New Aging

New Aging

Live smarter now to live better forever
By **Matthias Hollwich** *with* Bruce Mau Design

PENGUIN BOOKS
An imprint of Penguin Random House LLC
375 Hudson Street
New York, New York 10014
penguin.com

Library of Congress Cataloging-in-Publication Data

Names: Hollwich, Matthias, author. | Krichels, Jennifer, author.
Title: New aging : live smarter now to live better forever / Matthias
    Hollwich, Jennifer Krichels.
Description: New York : Penguin Books, 2016.
Identifiers: LCCN 2015048425 | ISBN 9780143128106 (paperback)
Subjects: LCSH: Older people. | Older people—Health and hygiene. | Older
    people—Dwellings. | Aging. | BISAC: SELF-HELP / Aging. | PSYCHOLOGY /
    Developmental / Adulthood & Aging. | HOUSE & HOME / Design & Construction.
Classification: LCC HQ1061 .H567 2016 | DDC 305.26—dc23

Printed in the United States of America
10 9 8 7 6 5 4 3 2 1

Designed by Bruce Mau Design

Author: Matthias Hollwich *with* Jennifer Krichels
Design: Bruce Mau Design | brucemaudesign.com
Hunter Tura, Tom Keogh, Cristian Ordóñez,
Elvira Barriga, and Kaila Jacques
Illustration: Robert Samuel Hanson

Dedication This book is in honor of Barbara and Walter Hollwich, and my grandmothers, Omi, Mausi, and grandaunt, Uschi. Thank you to the University of Pennsylvania for the opportunity to teach your students about aging and architecture, and to Robert Kasirer for the opportunity to work on BOOM, an ~~retirement~~ empowerment community. Thank you Marc Kushner for being the best business partner in the world. Thank you James Roebuck for putting up with me coming home late and writing throughout weekends.

Table of Contents

Why New Aging

When I turned forty, I realized that, according to current statistics, I had lived about half of my life. Curious about my future, I started researching aging. I was interested to learn what society and architecture have to offer to make sure the next half of my life is fulfilled and happy.

I didn't like what I was seeing.

Starting with research and design at the University of Pennsylvania and my architectural office, Hollwich Kushner Architecture (HWKN), I tasked students, faculty, architects, and researchers to come up with new and progressive ideas that could make aging a fulfilling process. The results were amazing: a retirement community could become an empowerment environment, a nursing home could turn into a healthiness hub, an informal volunteering app could provide support to older people. All very visionary ideas, but we realized that it would take decades to implement these visions as designers, and doing it one building at a time was just not fast enough.

This is why I started to write *New Aging*, a book that takes everything I have learned about aging and how society, architecture, and cities can perform better, and breaks it down into simple principles and actions that all of us can take today and every day —so we can live smarter now to live better forever—personally and as a society.

Matthias Hollwich

Live Smarter Now to Live Better Forever

New Aging is an eye-opening guide to life, offering easily implementable steps that have a positive effect on our long-term future.

This process begins with developing a new attitude toward aging: Expanding our social reach by inviting friends into our family circle, finding new ways to stay relevant to the world around us, adopting habits for staying fit and eating well, experimenting with transportation alternatives to using a car, looking at our homes with a new eye (and then changing our living spaces if needed), and enlisting the services that will guarantee our independence far into the future.

We can implement this blueprint all at once or step by step throughout the years. Yes, there are hurdles that we have to overcome in life, especially when getting older, but we have the opportunity to take small, almost playful actions to remove these hurdles even before they become an issue. Once removed, they are not just gone for us; with our lives as an example, they can also be removed for our families, friends, and neighbors so we all can live the life we want, all life long.

And this is how you do it.

New Aging

1

Love Aging

Imagine taking everything we associate with aging, from the loss of freedom and vitality to boredom, and throwing it out the window. These ideas are products of a society that has not yet cracked the code of aging. What if we as a society decided to transform our fear of aging into an appreciation for the beauty of living? A positive attitude toward aging is a start and will allow us to enjoy every bit of the journey. Since one of the principles of longevity is a positive attitude toward life, it might even allow us to live longer.

Aging is a gift, a once-in-a-lifetime opportunity. As we age, we have the chance to make sure that every day counts and that we can live the life we want, all life long. The sum of a lifetime of days lived well is more valuable than any other thing in the world. It's also a gift you can give the people around you, so that they will learn these lessons early through the examples you set.

Aging Is a gift.

Give yourself the gift of living in the moment, and start each day with at least one very special experience: eat a delicious meal, meet a beloved friend, learn something new, or buy yourself a treat.

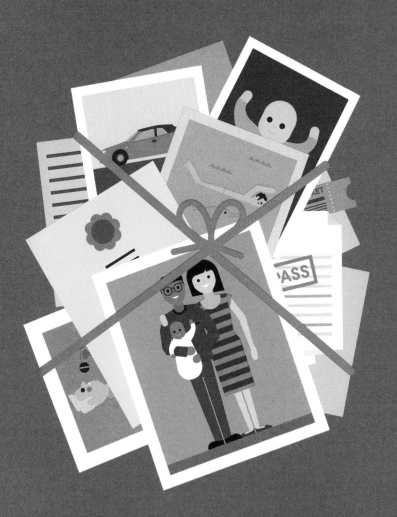

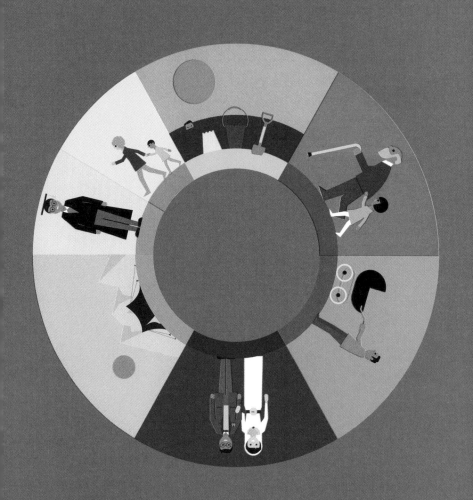

Through the passage of birth and adolescence to early adulthood and the point of reaching maturity with wisdom and calmness, every stage of life is a moment to visit with open eyes, like traveling to a new country. No matter our location, we can be explorers in our own lives by welcoming a sense of the unknown throughout life. Curiosity is the key to triggering a desire to explore and experience more.

Take the Trip of a Lifetime.

Try something new this week, from the simple—like reorganizing a part of your home or visiting a new part of your town—to something more dramatic—like swimming, gardening, or stargazing.

Aging needs to be met with a sense of adventure! Approaching life changes with wonder instead of anxiety lets us be curious and excited about the future. When we are young, we have an easy time tapping into qualities like optimism, curiosity, and openness to new ideas, but there's no reason we can't nurture this instinct and carry it through every stage of life. Every time you feel trepidation or reluctance, remember the tangible effect that a new experience can have on your life: better health, increased lifespan, more lively social surroundings, and a better quality of life.

Don't Worry, Be Adventurous.

Write down the ten things you most want to experience this year. Begin to envision what you would need to do to make just one of these dreams happen.

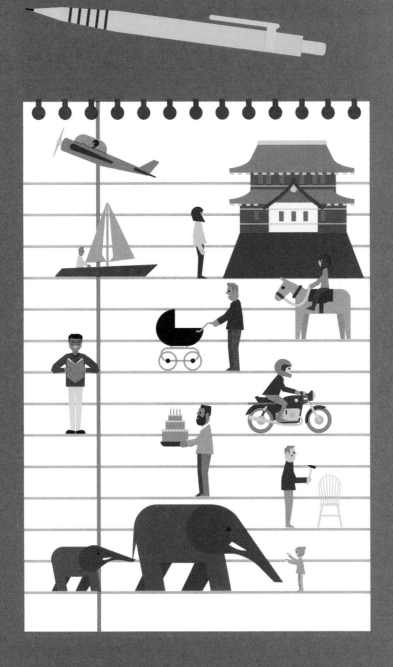

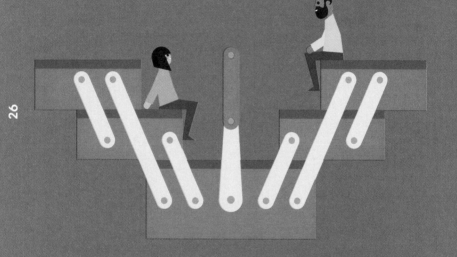

In the beginning of life, we only know how to eat and drink. Over time, our abilities multiply, with skills added daily. Some may be brand-new activities that broaden our horizons, while others may be repeated practices that deepen our mastery of one thing. Still others may be opportunities to grow and triumph during times of adversity. Aging allows us to accumulate a wealth of experience that defines who we are.

Collect a Set of Tools.

Make a list of the ten most influential talents you've developed in your lifetime, and share them with your family and friends so they can learn them, too.

Remember when you first used the Internet? Experiencing the transformation of our society is fascinating, and it is a privilege to take part in progress in the arts, science, and social issues. But we can also participate in the story. No matter what part of history we were first conscious of, whether the fight for civil rights or the election of the first African-American president or the advent of our digitally connected society, we can find countless ways to have conversations and become active in current movements.

Participate in History Being Made.

Think about the most interesting things going on today and participate on a local, national, or even international scale. Consume the news, volunteer at a political campaign, or lead an initiative to build a new monument in your town.

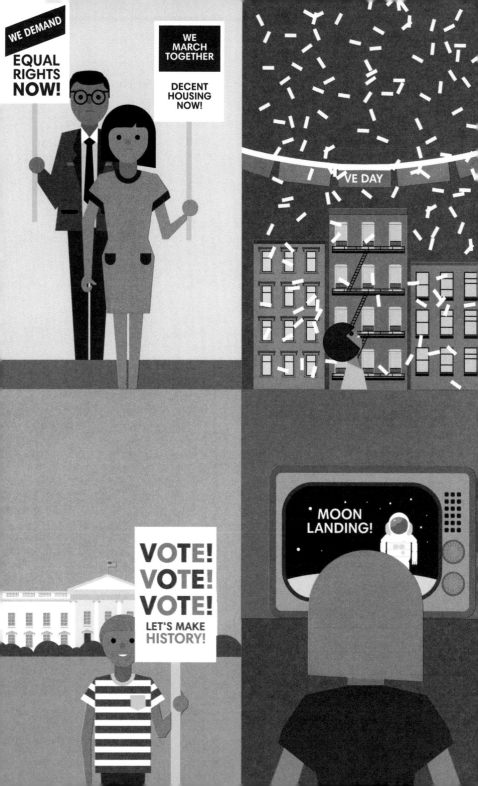

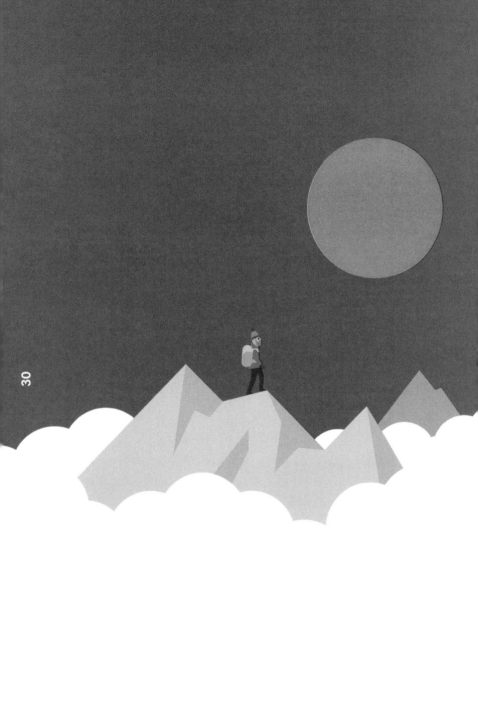

The older we get, the more we approach unknown territory. However, we should replace the word *old* with the term *pioneer*. We are the vanguard, pushing the depth of human experience to the next threshold. We've earned the freedom to explore the rest of our life without limits and hesitations. We can do things we never dreamed before.

Be a Pioneer.

A pioneer is expected to explore new ground. What is the one thing you always wanted to change about the world around you? Now is the time to voice it, and change it.

Let's face it: There are no "old people" in the world. There's only you and me a few years from now. We will have aged, but we are still the same people, only with more experience. Each of us knows more now than we did a minute ago.

Don't Discriminate Against Yourself.

Never call anybody "elderly," and never be angry that the person in front you might be a bit slower. It is human nature to slow down. Take a breath and remember to live in the moment.

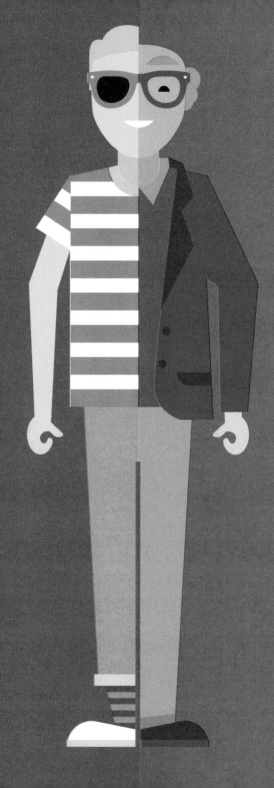

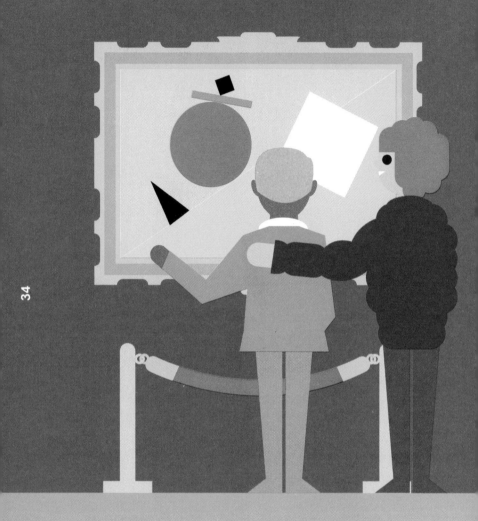

Don't miss a chance to walk in the shoes of an older person. Many of us encounter the process of getting older for the first time through our families, and we can learn a lot about aging through older family members. Helping them with important tasks and decisions is not only fulfilling, but also a learning experience that allows us to grow and develop our own attitudes toward aging in the future.

Take Aging for a Test Drive.

Pick up the phone and call the oldest person you know. Talk about their experience with aging and how they deal with it on a day-by-day basis.

2

Be Social

We are social by nature, and everybody needs diverse relationships with family, close friends, colleagues, and casual acquaintances. Healthy friendships are important, both physically and psychologically, to our overall well-being. As we age, the social network becomes even more important. It is our safety net. Staying social will allow us to invest in our community, stay current on events, and meet new people. Today, it is easier than ever to expand our ideas of what constitutes our inner circle. Expand yours—it is an investment in the future.

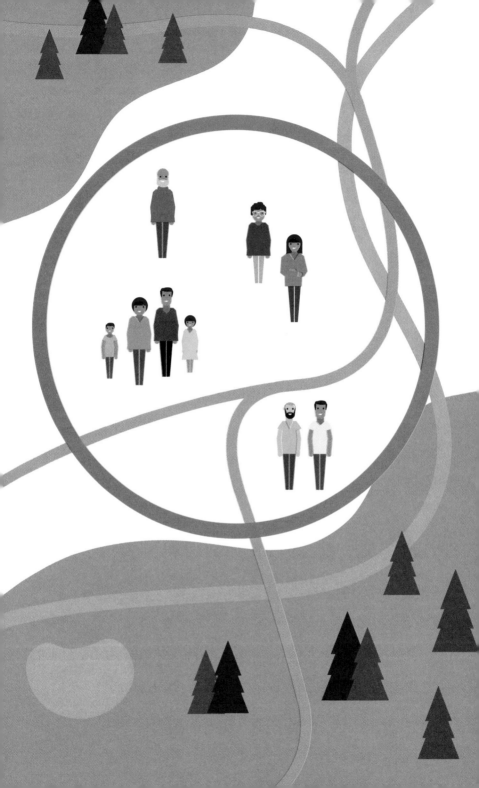

Family is important to social health at any stage in life. It's more obvious during our earliest years, when we live under one roof. Though we might move to a different city or country as we find our own relationships, we have to keep in mind that proximity is the key to allowing family members to watch out for one another. When we consider a move later in life, we should plan on moving closer—calibrating the distance so that everyone is spread out enough to enjoy independence, but close enough to be able to look out for one another regularly.

Get Closer.

Take a map and circle where your closest family members and friends live, then consider how, in the future, you can live closer.

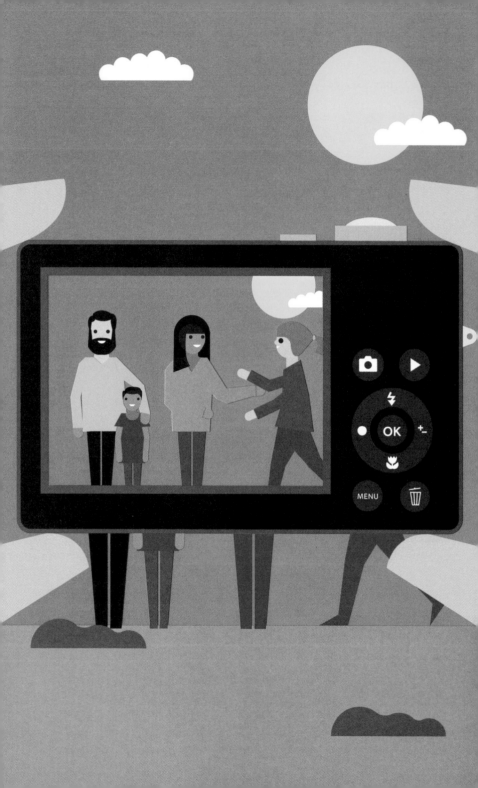

Modern life has transformed traditional family structures—the people we consider family are not necessarily blood relatives. We have redefined what family is, expanding the definition by inviting other kinds of relationships into our inner circle and ultimately enriching our lives and sense of security.

Treat Best Friends Like Family.

Think of your three best friends and start considering them your siblings. Begin new family traditions with them and include them in holiday celebrations and special occasions.

During our adult lives, we spend the majority of our working days with colleagues and collaborators. But we can include them in our inner circle beyond work as well, creating meaningful friendships that will last longer than the job. Colleagues offer a wealth of connections we can tap into, creating a social "glue" around us; we already have synchronized interests and common lifestyles, thanks to our work. Because of these shared experiences and professional goals, former colleagues might also be instrumental in launching independent ventures down the line—imagine the potential of working with friends we trust to build something new.

Turn Colleagues into Friends and Partners.

Make plans to meet with your closest colleagues after work this week and start integrating them into your inner circle.

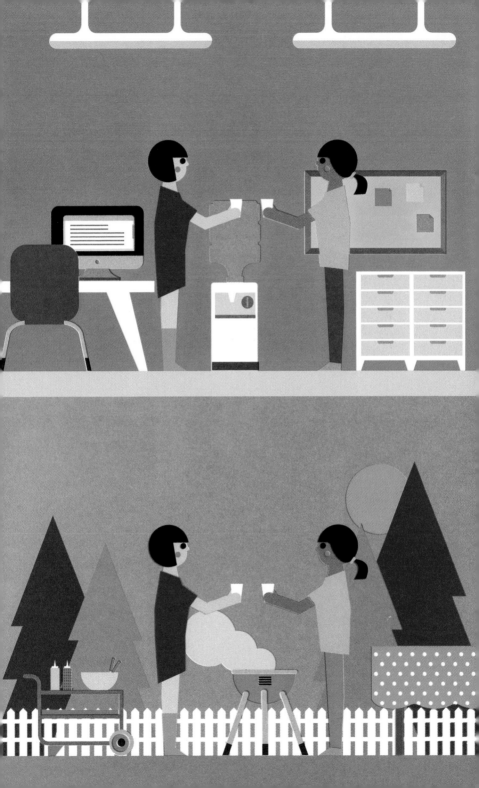

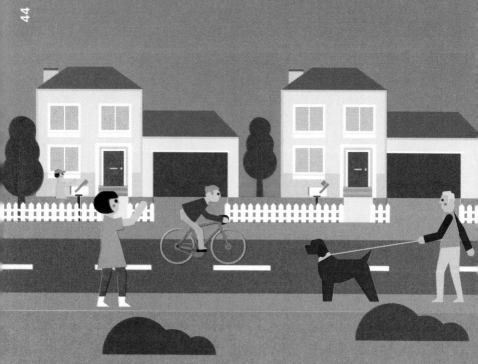

We already have our communities in common, so why not look locally for new friends whose homes are close by, or who frequent the same newsstand every Sunday morning? The easiest way to start making neighborhood friends is to get out of the house, say hello, and participate in local activities. Once acquainted, we can initiate conversations while checking the mail, synchronize weekly trips to the market, and offer information and assistance to newcomers. Think of being immersed in our communities as a gift that keeps giving. We'll be more connected with local events and more likely to find fulfilling day-to-day activities.

Meet the Neighbors.

The next time you see your neighbors, exchange email addresses and phone numbers and get in touch periodically, especially when it's been a while since you ran into each other on the street.

We shouldn't leave our neighborhoods to chance—we can encourage our friends to live close by. Ties among inhabitants enrich a neighborhood exponentially by creating more support for local businesses and centers of activity, not to mention making life more lively in general. Imagine being able to bump into your favorite people close to home! Whether in a suburb or apartment building, we can actively recruit our friends to the neighborhood to build a stronger community.

Good Friends Make Great Neighborhoods.

Invite your friends over for a walk around your neighborhood, pointing out all the special things about the area. Pitch the idea of living closer to one another.

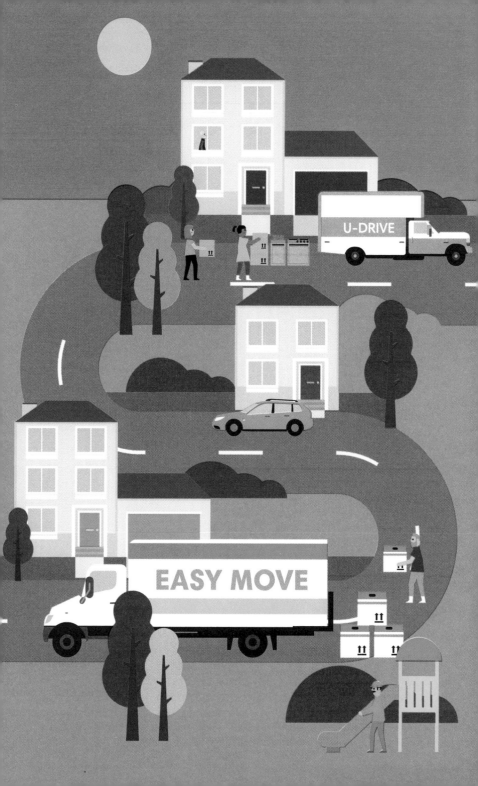

Remember sharing a dorm with other students in college? For many of us, this was the most social living experience of our lives. We can learn from the good aspects of dorm living, like shared costs, mutual accountability, and built-in fun, and apply them to our future living arrangements by becoming housemates. But because we are adults (and the joy of dorm living only goes so far), we have to consider home upgrades that will make this arrangement more feasible; multiple entrances into the home, private master bedrooms and baths, and numerous social areas for individual enjoyment are key to making this setup work.

Housemates Are the New Roommates.

Review the layout of your home and explore the opportunity to share it with a close friend in the future.

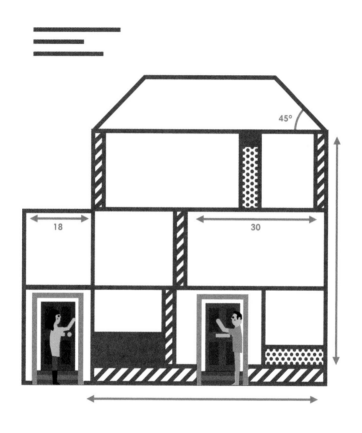

Breaking down the fences between our house and our neighbors' will create an open flow between properties. We can share our pool and lawn so that we can enjoy our neighbors' sundecks and grills in return. Removing traditional barriers between homes helps make our community more social, while allowing everyone to enjoy more amenities than we would alone. What we lose in exclusivity we gain in social connectivity.

Breaking Down Fences Makes Great Neighbors.

Organize a neighborhood meeting at which everybody presents their special amenity that can be shared, and start breaking down barriers—ideologically or even literally—one fence at a time.

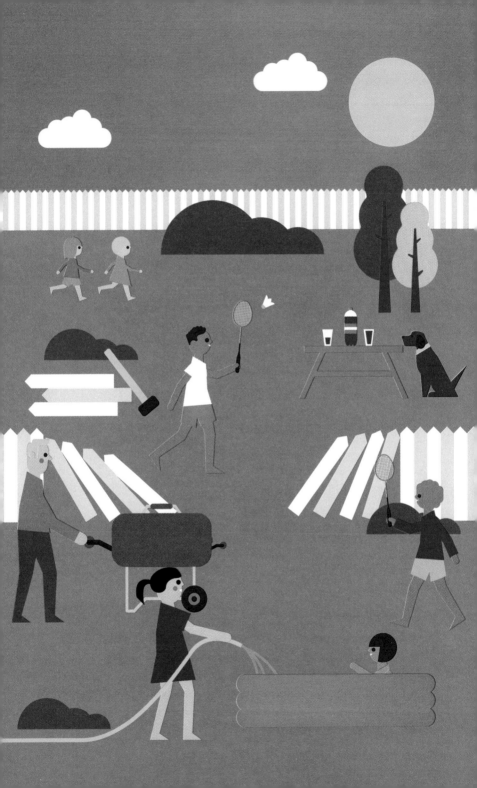

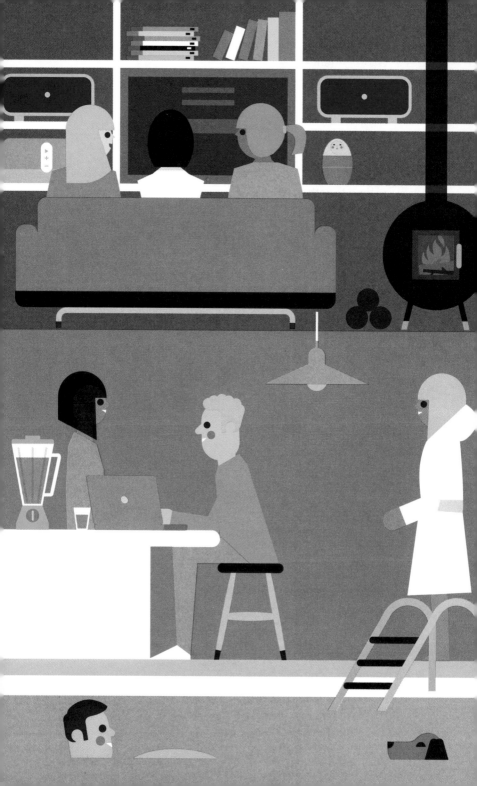

To keep your home lively and your social life active, work to attract visitors to your residence, making sure their visit is fun and not a burden for anyone. While there's a benefit to scaling down, we should consider creating living spaces that have easy access to amenities that are important to our social lives: for example, a pool, sauna, Wi-Fi, an inviting kitchen, or a playroom can make even a normal day exciting. Such state-of-the-art amenities will give you and guests the ultimate "staycation" and encourage everyone to spend more time together. Once our homes are attractive for others, they are more attractive for us.

Turn Your Home into a Clubhouse.

Review your home and add at least one unique and fun amenity that will reward you and those who visit.

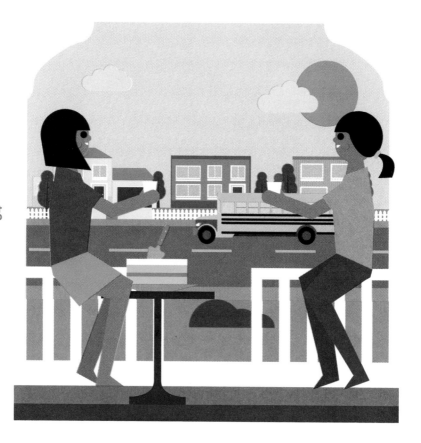

Historically, the porch was a place to enjoy the privacy of a house while having contact with neighbors. By adding comfortable front porches or stoops to our homes, we carry on this tradition. We can create alternative "porches" or places of gathering, too. In an apartment, don't lock yourself in and watch TV—open the door to invite neighbors in whenever the mood strikes. Consider the hallway Main Street and the front of the building as an interface with the community.

Make Your Porch a Front-Row Seat.

Hold an open house this weekend: open your front door for a day, add a sign that reads "Welcome In," and share some refreshments. You might be surprised how social your neighborhood is.

Adding a friend to our activities allows us to share our experiences and create stronger ties with the people we know. It gives them the opportunity to join a new activity, meet people, and become a bigger part of our lives. The reverse is true as well—it's a great feeling to accept an invite to something different. We should be open to our friends including us in new experiences.

Do It Together.

Think of your daily tasks and how each could become something you do with a companion. Call a friend to join whatever you do today.

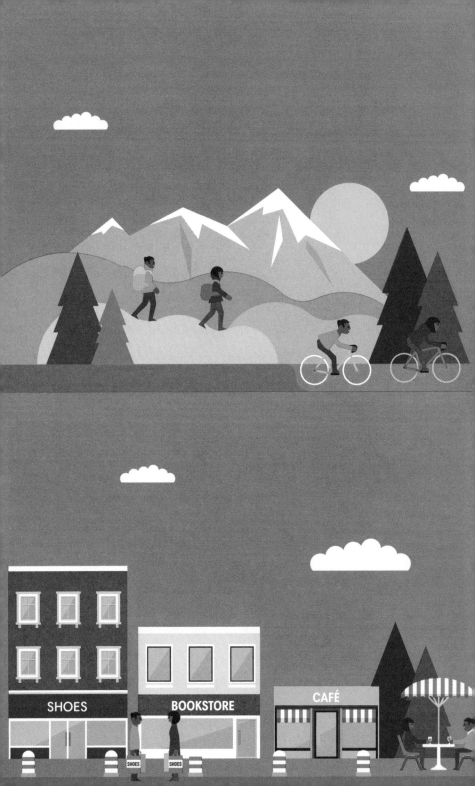

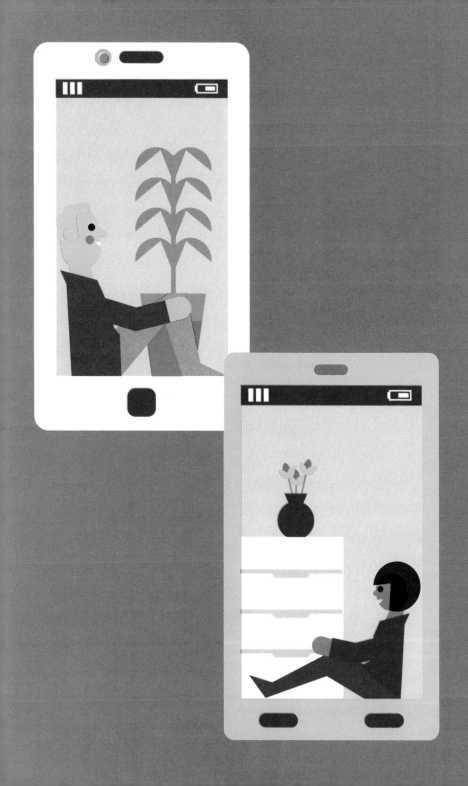

Prioritize friendships, and be proactive about maintaining them. Don't sit at home and wait for the phone to ring—cultivate these relationships by scheduling regular social activities, like a biweekly lunch with coworkers, a Saturday-morning stroll with a neighbor, or a weekend getaway with friends. Catching up doesn't have to take long when done regularly. Scheduling a fifteen-minute block of time each day to write a letter or phone someone we care about can help us feel more connected.

Phone a Friend.

Get in touch with three people today and make plans to get together with them this month.

It is easy to just go on with life and concentrate on all the tasks that we have to accomplish on a daily basis. But let's not forget that there is more to life, like sharing experiences in person. We can make a rule to be social at least twice a week, by meeting with friends or family and choosing an activity that everybody will enjoy: shared dinners, shopping, museum visits, or sporting events. We can also dedicate specific days for social activities or to be spontaneous. Once we begin to involve more people in our lives, they will start involving us in theirs.

Make a Rule to Be Social.

Review your weekly schedule and explore how you can add other people to it. Use a shared online calendar so that people can RSVP easily to group events.

Aug 21

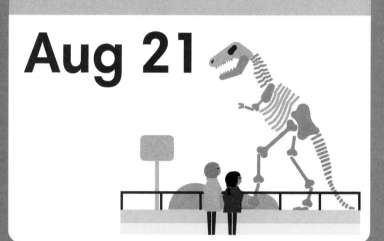

Aug 22

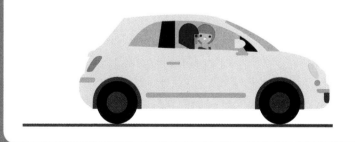

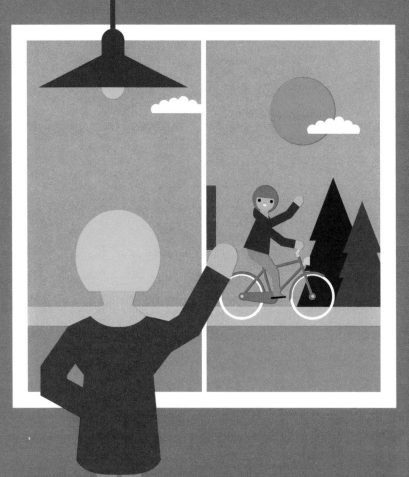

We can keep our social engines running by fostering opportunities for encounters that nurture our relationships. When looking for a place to live, we should look for a home surrounded by public places where we can meet friends or acquaintances, whether intentionally or spontaneously.

See and Be Seen.

Plan a daily walk that includes farmers' markets, parks, playgrounds, and cafés—all of which are likely places to bump into people.

The ways in which we organize our lives have been completely changed by digital technology. And so have our schedules. In today's highly planned world, finding a feasible way to organize commitments is crucial to enjoying life. From fixed long-term appointments to spontaneous get-togethers that can happen "on demand," we have to make sure that we are not left off the agenda. Traditional calendars are now less useful. Take advantage of new online social management tools and allow people to join individual activities without long-term commitment to a group.

Advertise Your Schedule.

Go online today and use social media to set up face-to-face ways to socialize in real life.

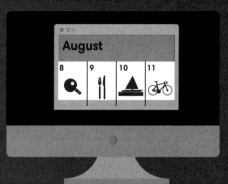
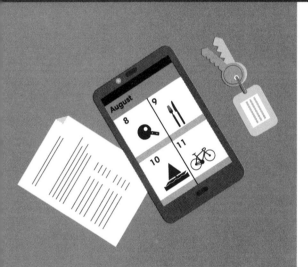
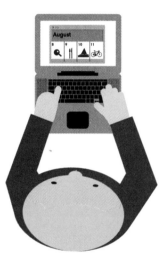
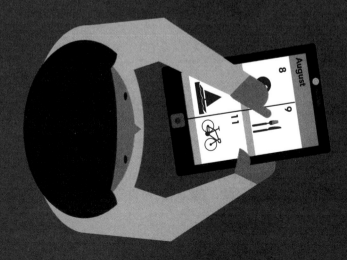

3

Never Retire

Retirement is one of the worst ideas our society has invented. Some of us may be sick of our jobs and looking forward to quitting—but we shouldn't wait for retirement to do so. Instead, we should quit the jobs we never liked in the first place and start ones that are fulfilling in the long run. There are countless reasons to continue working in some capacity, the most important of which is longevity. Doing activities that are meaningful to us can extend our life expectancies.

Rather than retiring, consider working part-time or on a contract basis. Many employers will welcome the opportunity to have our knowledge still on hand. Explore ways of creating a flexible schedule by consulting independently, telecommuting, or using flextime while staying active in the workforce. Online freelancing platforms have also opened up opportunities to tap into part-time work. Broadcast your freelance services and see if any attractive projects come your way. This will leave you connected to your professional community and may lead to larger business advancements and networking opportunities while freeing up time to explore other interests.

Find an Alternative to Quitting.

Create a list of your core strengths, those that could contribute to new ventures, and think about where you can apply these assets at work and beyond.

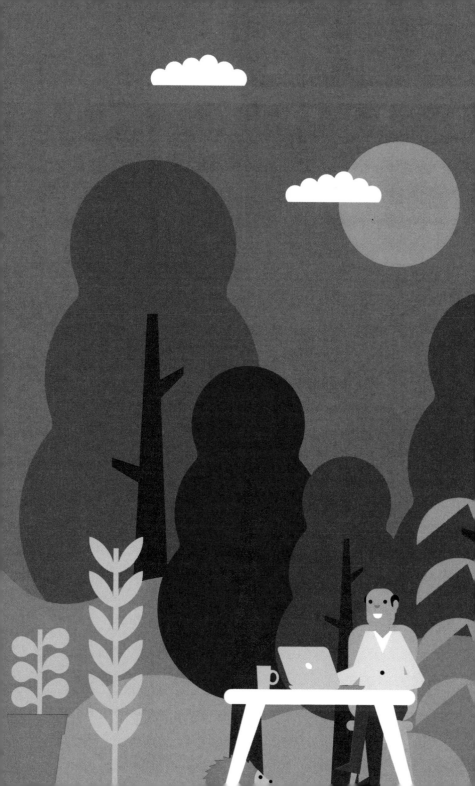

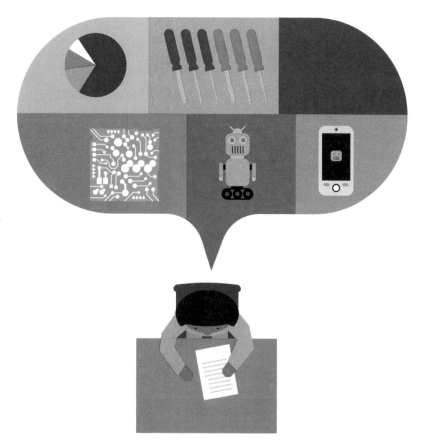

If we choose to retire from our old job, we can move on and use our own creativity to build our next career. Take a note from the foundational legends of entrepreneurs everywhere and start a company from the garage, living room, or coffee shop down the street. Starting a business later in life gives us many advantages, including years of experience and management history on which to build. Once we are "retired," our time and networks of potential clients and partners are assets that can be put to work right away. Starting a company without the immediate pressure of success gives us leeway to cultivate real innovation while doing what we always wanted to do.

Start-Up Your Life.

Start writing an elevator pitch for your dream company and think about ways to start it. Once you're done with your elevator pitch, expand it into a business plan.

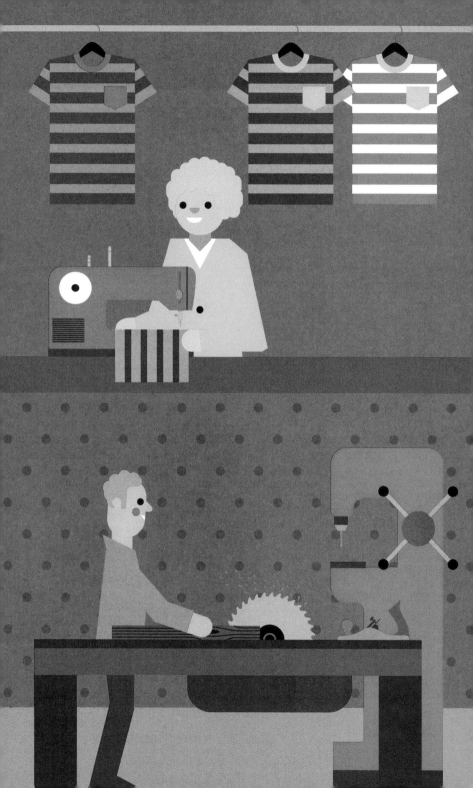

Consider the things we do in our leisure time, childhood passions that went dormant in middle age, natural abilities that have been forgotten, or the networking ability that a previous career has given us. Can any of these be leveraged into a slower-paced second career? A quilting enthusiast can start a side business at a local craft fair or online marketplace. A great cook can give neighborhood cooking classes on brilliant thirty-minute dinner recipes.

Put Hobbies to Work.

A former high school soccer star can sign up to referee the neighborhood league. Even something as simple as a love for children can be channeled into part-time work at a day-care center. Continue to be a contributing member of society. Transforming one or two passions into fulfilling jobs could add a new dimension to life.

Make a list of your favorite hobbies and think about how you could turn one of them into a viable business:

Arranging flowers.

Car maintenance.

Carpentry.

Coaching.

Decorating.

Tourism.

Nothing is more life affirming than giving back. When we do good for our fellow citizens, we connect to a wider community. Volunteering is a great way to meet other people, gain recognition, discover purpose, and develop a sense of ownership in society. We can find opportunities that align with our interests and schedules through local volunteer resource centers, or we can volunteer help within our social networks.

Give a Little, Gain a Lot.

Look up places to volunteer in your neighborhood today, and select the one you feel most passionate about.

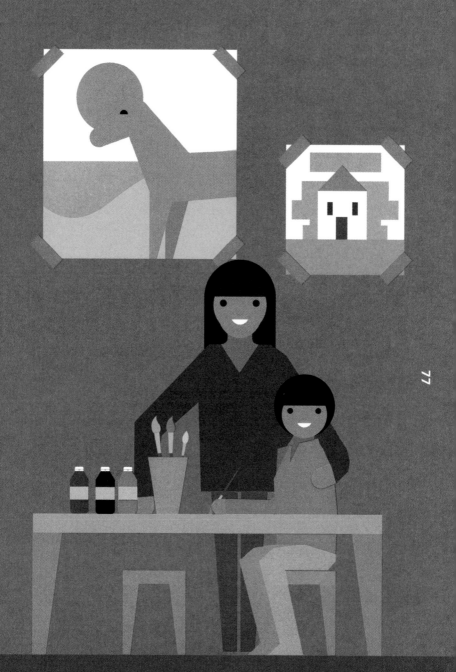

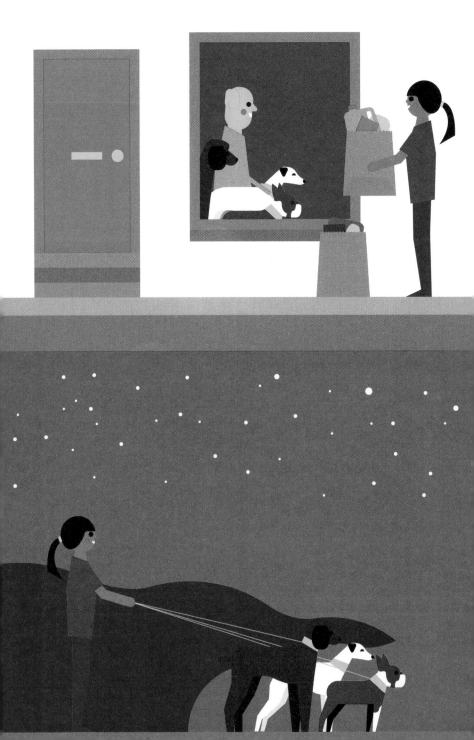

When we have free time on our hands, we can participate in the day-to-day life of our families, whether it's babysitting for grandchildren, taking care of older family members, or helping with household tasks and errands. If we approach this like a "real" job, we can also begin to think of ways to excel: creating more family activities, running an efficient social calendar, and saving money for others—all while getting out of the house ourselves.

Be Generous with Time.

Call your closest family members and friends and ask them what type of help would benefit them the most. Look at your own life and determine what you can ask for help with, too.

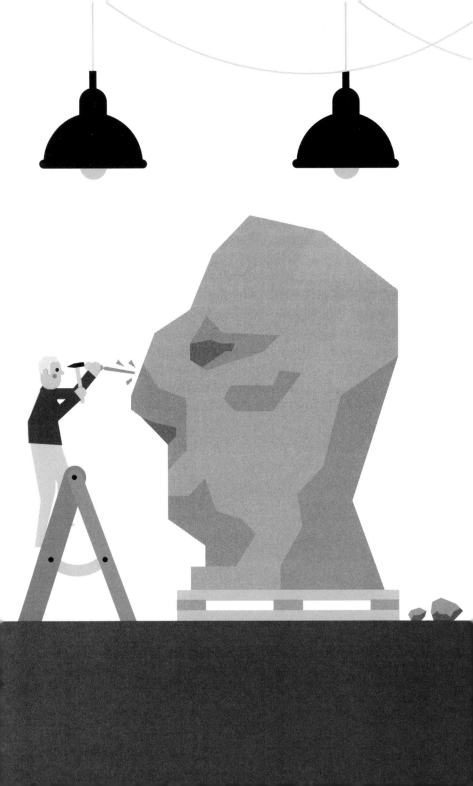

Taking classes for fun when there is nothing at stake beyond self-improvement is far more enjoyable than the required classes from our school days. Continuing education keeps our minds active and exposes us to intergenerational learning environments. Learn something new that could open up opportunities for work, volunteering, and other social contributions.

Be a Student Forever.

Look for the three closest educational opportunities in your area. Many colleges and universities will offer people in the community the option to audit classes. Study their offerings and sign up for at least one class next semester.

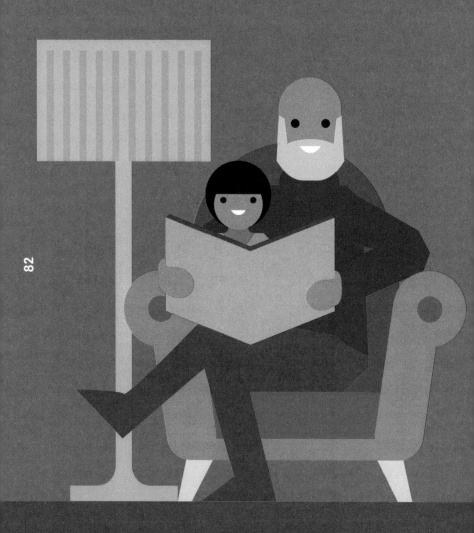

Once a president has left office, the work has just begun. For many, the next phase of life involves preserving what they know by preparing the presidential library and writing a book, or by starting philanthropic organizations and speaking at institutions. We, too, can record our experiences so that they can be meaningful in the future. Personal history is worth preserving as a contribution to a broader historical context, and as a bridge between generations. Doing this ourselves allows us to curate what we are remembered for and pass along valuable information to those around us.

Preserve Your Heritage.

Start a blog, write in a journal, shoot a home movie, or record knowledge through an oral history project. Remember that our history is as important as our future.

When we join the rat race, we often start relying on services and purchase products that make our time manageable. To keep these expenses in check, we should reevaluate which of these we might be able to do ourselves once we have a freer schedule. Becoming a DIY-er keeps more money in our pockets while providing us with the opportunity to take pleasure in small, accomplishable tasks.

Do It Yourself.

This week, try cooking at home versus ordering out, cutting your own lawn, or tackling a home improvement project you know you can accomplish in less than a day. You may be surprised at how satisfying it is to do things yourself.

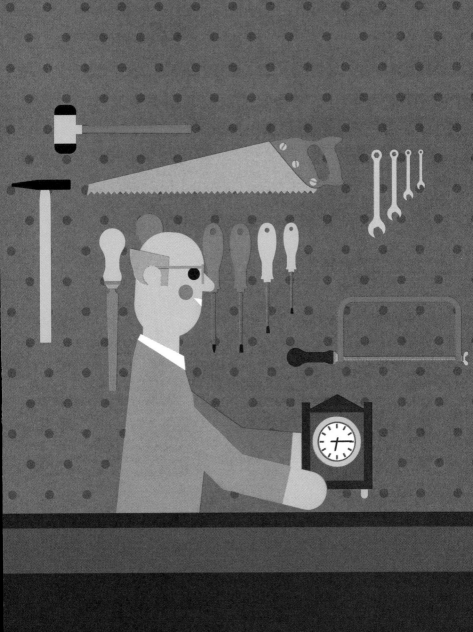

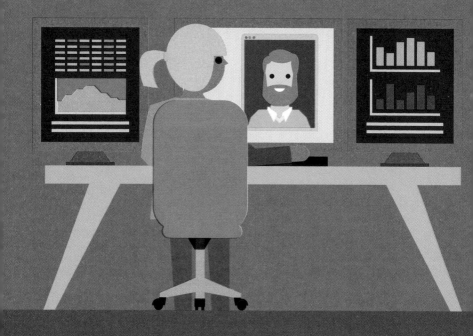

Being active in investment trading with small amounts of our funds allows us to stay informed about daily happenings, while reaping the financial benefits that come from smart decisions. Though funds should be managed conservatively when we're older, keeping part of our finances more active lets us directly participate in the economics of each day. Being a well-informed trader means staying current with world news—do this and you'll become an informed citizen in the process.

Become a Trader.

Pick up a business magazine and study today's top-performing companies. Follow them over the coming days, staying up to date on their progress. Use the knowledge to talk with your broker and to make sound investing decisions.

4

Stay Fit

Staying fit is a proven health and life extender—one that we can control. It is much easier to establish a fitness habit now than to fight off extra pounds and health complications later. This area of mainte-nance is highly influenced by our environment. If we place ourselves in settings that inspire us to participate in physical activities, we stand the best chance of enjoying the many benefits of fitness.

Most of us go to the gym to work out, but there are many ways to be active in our surrounding environments that are not explicitly labeled "exercise." Find alternative exercise opportunities within your neighborhood, whether it's walking up the longest set of stairs in the local mall, swimming in the public pool, strolling around the biggest museum, biking from one side of the city to the other, or cruising through every department in the department store. Consider getting from one place to another your chance to get a miniworkout. This even includes parking our cars a little farther from our destination or getting off the bus a few blocks before our stop.

Exercise Without Meaning To.

Each day this week, use a step counter to reach a goal. Turn on your creativity and explore the potential for exercise in your neighborhood. Every little bit counts: a daily fifteen-minute walk adds up to 5,475 minutes—almost one hundred hours—of walking a year!

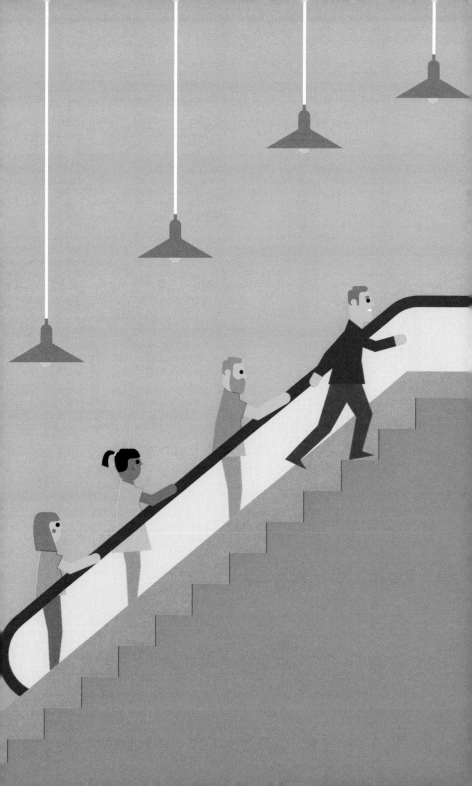

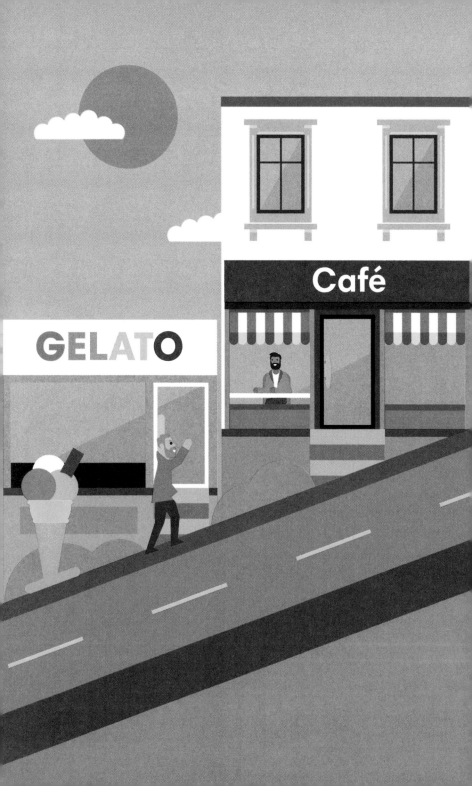

It is convenient to stay home—but inconvenience can add a healthy edge to our lives. Let's make sure we get out of the house, socialize with old friends, meet new people, collect fresh experiences, and exercise in the process. Remember that every time we leave the house we add a microexercise to our daily routine, burn calories, and breathe fresh air. Minimizing the use of cars lets us bike or walk more, take in the beauty of our surroundings, and meet other people.

Find Reasons to Get Out.

Look at this month's calendar and add a new reason to get out each day: drink a coffee in a café, see a game in person, visit a museum, shop at a market, watch a movie, or just go window-shopping.

Our houses have kitchens, living rooms, dining rooms, and bedrooms—but often no area dedicated to exercise. We might not have an entire extra room, but we can still add multifunctional workout space to our homes. A living room can become a temporary yoga room, a study can be enhanced with cardio equipment, adding a running, biking, or stepping machine. Our kitchens can turn into places to burn calories if we lift small weights while we watch the lasagna cook. We can use our bedrooms for stretching, push-ups, and crunches.

Turn Home into a Gym.

Turning your home into a gym will eliminate a lot of potential excuses for skipping a workout. Add three new exercises to your around-the-house routine this week, treating them as you would other essential parts of your day (like cooking, eating, and sleeping).

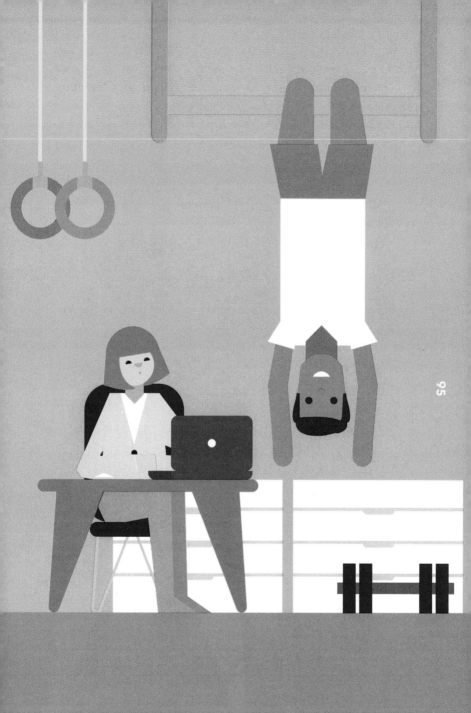

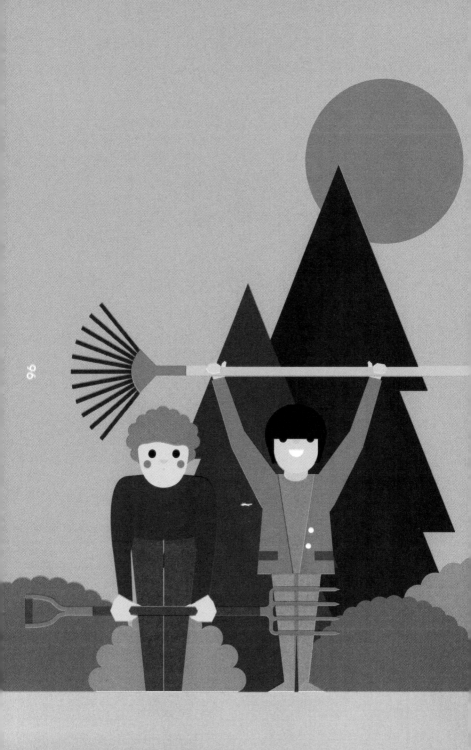

Instead of going to the gym, we can turn some of our leisure activities into opportunities to exercise. Rather than watching reruns, tune in to an exercise program or use a home entertainment system with fitness-focused video games. In real life, think of gardening as a way to build muscle strength and playing fetch with your dog as a great cardiovascular workout. Explore options for unconventional exercise: dance parties that happen in the morning and focus on wellness or scavenger hunts that transform entire cities into huge gaming fields.

Turn Workout Time into Playtime.

Look at your daily schedule and add a star next to any activity that could augment your traditional workout routine.

No matter the level at which we participate, sports are good ways to stay active and socially engaged while holding us accountable to a regular schedule. Whether it's basketball, rowing, biking, soccer playing, or tennis, joining a team inspires us to come back for more. Exercising with others adds a great social benefit to our workouts, and a little positive peer pressure ensures we keep up with our teammates. Even if you can no longer get out onto the ball field or tennis court, keep the social aspects of sports alive by attending a game with friends or watching one on TV with family.

Participate in the Social Aspect of Sports.

Call up your best friends and discuss sports that you can do together, so that you remind each other to stay fit and have fun while doing so.

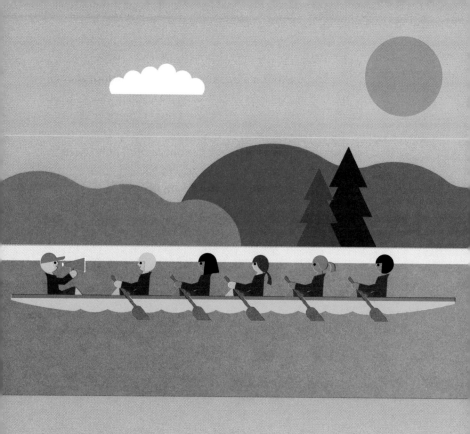
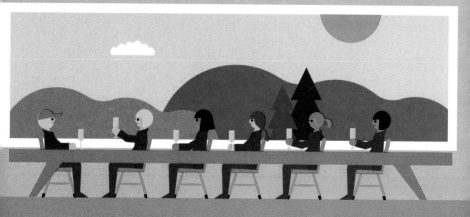

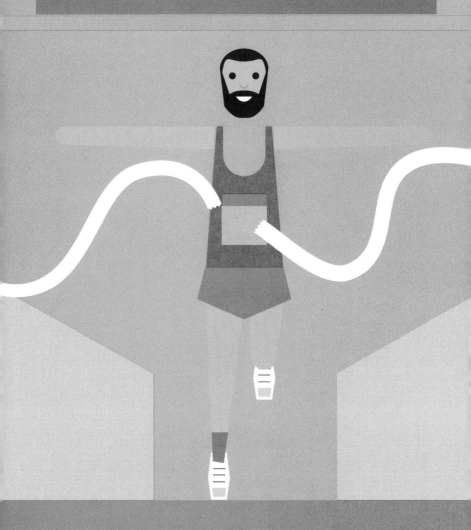

Being a professional in sports is not restricted to a certain age group. We can find an activity that we love and perform it at our best. From golfing, sailing, swimming, and fishing, to walking, biking, or tennis, there is always an opportunity to excel. Doing a sport professionally allows us to focus and set goals. It is a way to introduce more discipline and routine into life. Of course, there may be a time when professional activities will not be realistic, but we can aim for the best and let our bodies determine the rest. Being competitive has a motivating quality for us and those around us.

Become a Professional.

Pick your favorite sport and sign up for classes that will help you improve. Creating a goal will help you stick with it and, over time, help you to hone your skills.

When we try a new sport, we get momentum from the excitement of learning. As our skills improve, we can make a habit out of our new practice and over time we gain mental strength from trying new things and keeping our bodies active.

Find a New Activity to Create a New Opportunity.

Start with a list of athletic activities you have never done before and choose one to start.

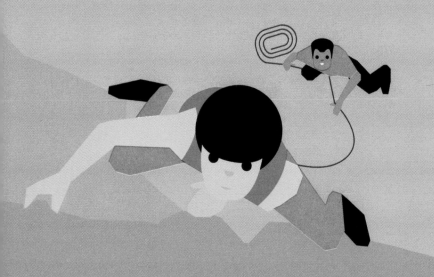

Try something new each day to keep the mind engaged as much as the body:

Check out the **local soft-ball** club.

Visit a **Tai Chi** class.

Take a **new walking route** every day for a month.

Join an **intra-mural league.**

Check out **an exercise class subscription** that gets you into new fitness studios in your city.

GYM

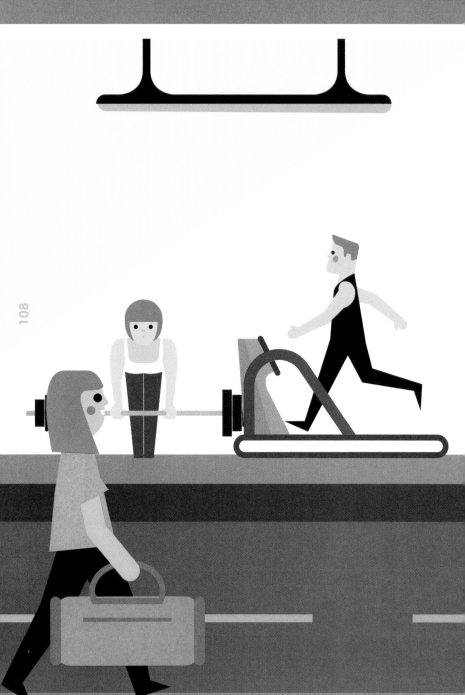

Visiting the gym is a wonderful opportunity to focus on strength and flexibility through activities that are offered within one location. Gyms also offer a familiar environment with standardized equipment and people to meet. The gyms we join should be close to home and attractive to work out in, providing more pleasure than pain and easily becoming part of our daily routines.

Go to the Gym.

If you don't have an active gym membership, sign up today. Find a place that makes you feel part of the club and gives you both physical and mental rewards.

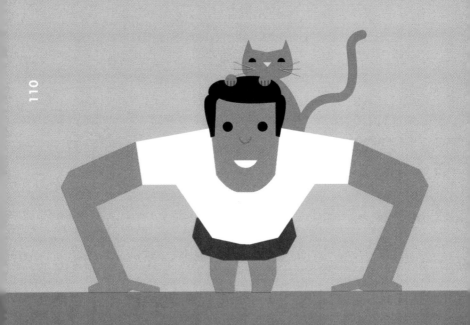

Whatever activity we pursue, we can do it with family or friends to keep our motivation high and our activity healthy. A workout partner can monitor our progress and vice versa. Even when doing individual activities like running or weight lifting, having someone to share benchmarks (or water breaks) with encourages us to stick to a routine even when our schedule is hectic or we feel like sleeping in.

Find a Workout Partner.

Go through your address book and convince your friends to meet twice a week for workouts, an athletic game, or a shared personal training session.

5

You Are How You Eat

A lot of books can help us reach nutritional goals—and they're helpful to read. *New Aging*, however, focuses on replacing snacking on the go with purposeful, healthy eating habits that create new experiences and bring people together. Since the beginning of time, food has united families and communities in cultures around the world. We can bring the act of eating into our lives in a way that enriches our relationships and our relationship to food at the same time. Food is greater than the sum of its ingredients.

In many cultures, it would be a sacrilege to scarf down a bag of chips on the run. Not only does eating slowly and mindfully help us eat less, it enhances the pleasure of the dining experience. Eating slowly helps us become more mindful of what we eat, and to get the appropriate relaxation that our bodies require.

Eat Slowly.

Sit down at a table three times a day; slow down, eat, and enjoy.

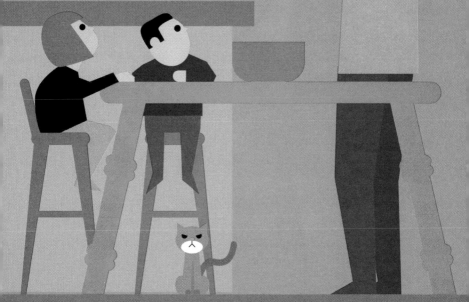

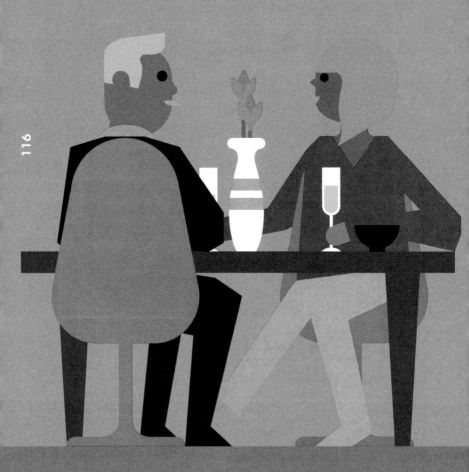

Remember that eating is about more than food. To master the art of eating in style, put on some music, light a few candles, turn off the TV and any other distractions, and concentrate on your meal. Eat at an actual table, and take time to decompress and appreciate every bite of food.

Eat in Style.

Make note of the things you like about your favorite restaurant and implement them at home.

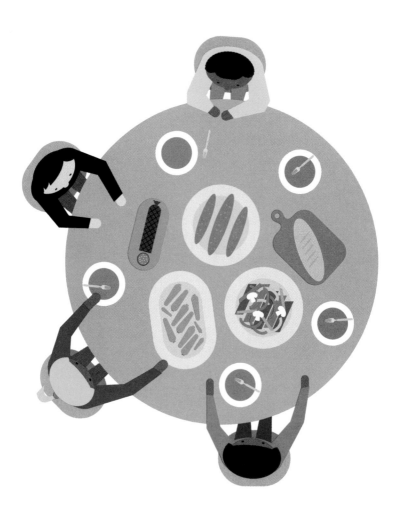

Eating with others encourages us to treat mealtime as an event worth savoring. It also makes us more conscious of what and how much we consume. Trade a formal dining room for a large kitchen with stools at the counter or other casual seating options so that friends and family can spontaneously drop by to chat and eat. This will make hosting informal lunches and dinners with friends easier to do on a regular basis.

Eat Social.

Set up your table in the center of the room and have at least four chairs around it. Call your friends and start eating together at least once a week.

Sometimes we watch a couple of cooking shows or read a magazine and feel like we need to cook a three-course meal every night of the week. But the reality of today's schedules is that people have less time to shop for groceries, let alone spend an hour or two (or five) on meal preparation and cleanup. Find ways to bring healthy ingredients into your home without breaking your back, whether by arranging for a delivery of produce and meat from local farms (or farm-share programs) or your nearby grocery store, or by tapping into the many Internet-based services that will send ingredients directly to your door.

Take It Easy.

Good food doesn't have to cost you your sanity. Cook a new, easy, healthy meal just once a week and expand your knowledge about how to make cooking convenient.

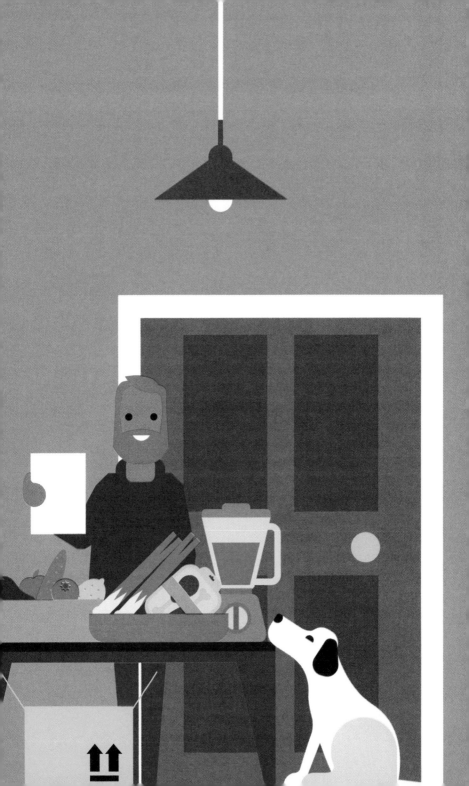

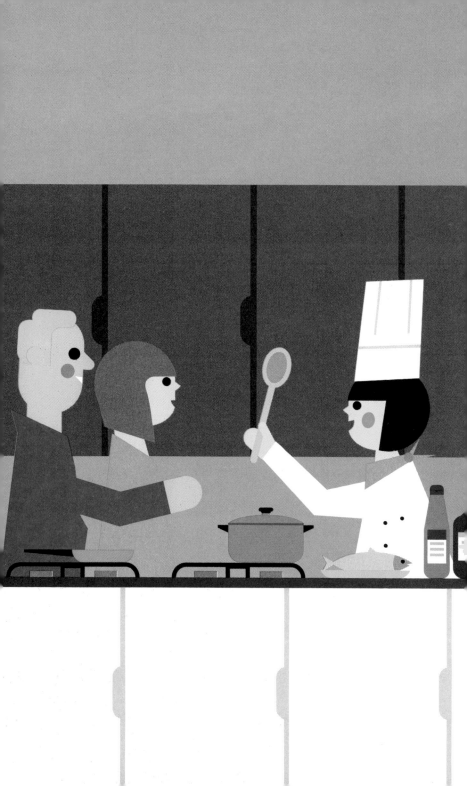

Picking up just a couple of new skills can take us from being kitchen novices to fledgling chefs. Cooking shows are great, but many community centers, private companies, and even the cooking store at the local mall offer classes and new recipes, as well as the opportunity for new social connections. We can also go the virtual route and add a tablet device to our kitchens so that cooking apps and videos are within reach at all times.

Learn from a Pro.

Show off new cooking skills to friends this week and share your new-found culinary knowledge with them.

Look for a local restaurant that serves good-quality food, and become a regular there. Reserve a communal table for weekly meetings, book a room for your birthday every year, and get to know the chef and staff. Supporting a local business will inject resources into an establishment that will, in turn, enhance the whole neighborhood. With regular patronage, local bars and cafés can be wonderful meeting places for the community, and often host musical acts and other entertainment, giving us the chance to meet diners while receiving great service.

Food Network.

Visit your favorite restaurant today and ask if you can set up a weekly table for yourself, your neighbors, and your friends.

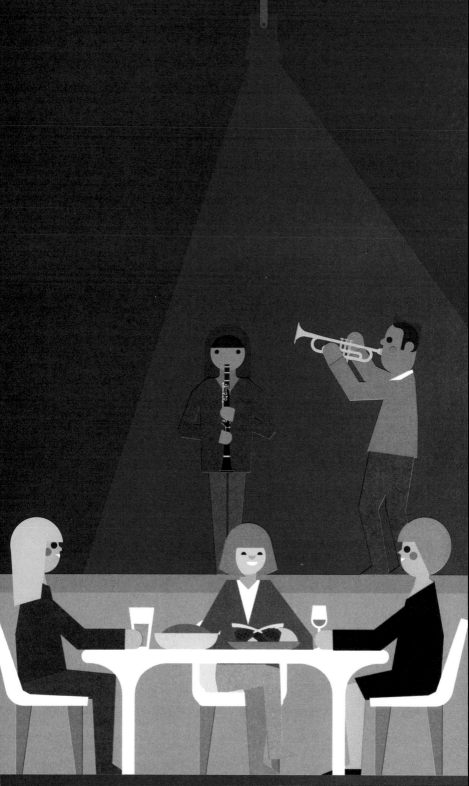

6

Access vs. Mobility

Mobility is a key feature in our lives. We like to travel and we have to move around to take care of daily needs and have pleasurable experiences. But at some point in our lives, mobility is harder to maintain. We might lose the ability to use our own cars or even walk around the block. This is why it is important to replace the idea of mobility with the idea of access—having a way to interact with the world and physically access the things we need and want ensures our quality of life remains intact.

Most of us need cars to get around. But what if we live in a city where everything is within walking distance? In that case, we can manage our lives without depending on our ability to drive. In an ideal scenario we can take care of our daily routine with a twenty-minute walk, and meet friends and neighbors on our way. If that is not the case we have three choices: move to a more urban location, work with the city and local retailers to diversify the options in the area, or pair up with friends and neighbors and find alternative ways to get around. Many private companies and community centers offer ride-sharing services and coordination for carpooling, which are oftentimes available at highly discounted rates or even at no cost at all. Enhancing our transportation approach with walking or biking is also a wonderful way to test out a "car-lite" existence while including exercise in our daily routines.

Make Your Car a Luxury.

Evaluate whether you live in a place where a car is a luxury or a necessity. Don't use your car for a week and explore all kinds of alternative options to stay mobile.

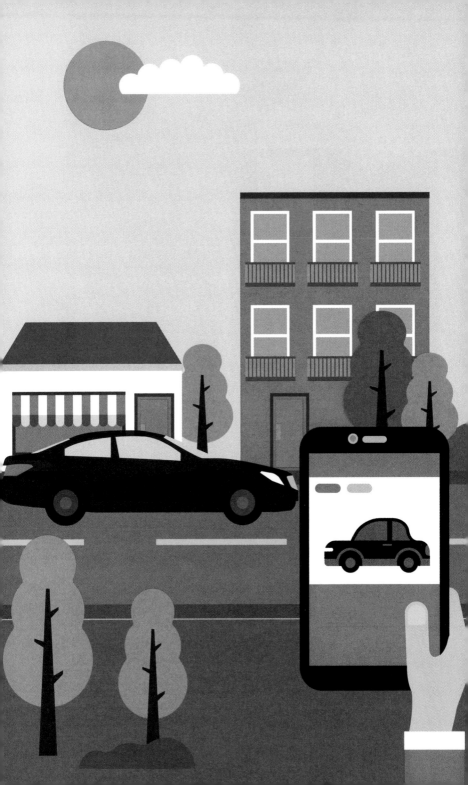

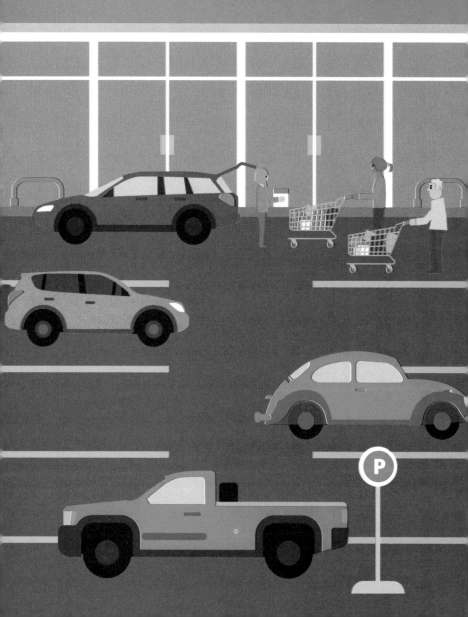

Why would you actually drive to a grocery store by yourself when you can do it with neighbors or friends and have fun on the way? Arrange for a dedicated driver who creates a route to key shopping destinations, and take care of your needs while enjoying the company of a group. Having a willing and able driver relieves stress for the nondrivers, and doing it together is helpful and fun. You might, in the process, even discover ways to share goods or bulk purchases. Ride-sharing is the future: it's good for the environment, costs less, and frees you up to enjoy the ride.

Pool Your Ride.

Organize a driving pool with your friends and neighbors and commit to a shared driving schedule. Switch up the responsibility and make sure it's fun.

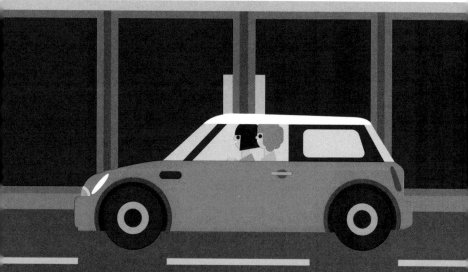

Research shows that the average car is only driven four percent of the time, while it costs about $9,000 each year—money we could all use for something else. Consider using a professional driver, eliminating worry about traffic or directions. Ordering a taxi, private car, or ride-share through an app has become common for many New York City residents, and is gaining popularity in other urban areas as well. By tapping into the driving services near us, we keep the advantages of car travel and enjoy a bit of luxury along the way.

Let Others Drive You.

Sign up for on-demand driving services today and use them exclusively for a week to evaluate their convenience and cost.

Why drive a car when the car can drive you? It may seem like science fiction now, but many companies are working on self-driving cars and other automated forms of transportation that could revolutionize the way we get around. For example, just nine thousand automated cars could replace every cab in New York City. Let's embrace the new technology and help governments and companies overcome regulatory challenges so we can add a promising solution to our living strategy in the near future.

Embrace the Self-Driving Car.

Sign up for news about self-driving cars and learn how you can support technology that will provide mobility and independence to people like us a few years from now.

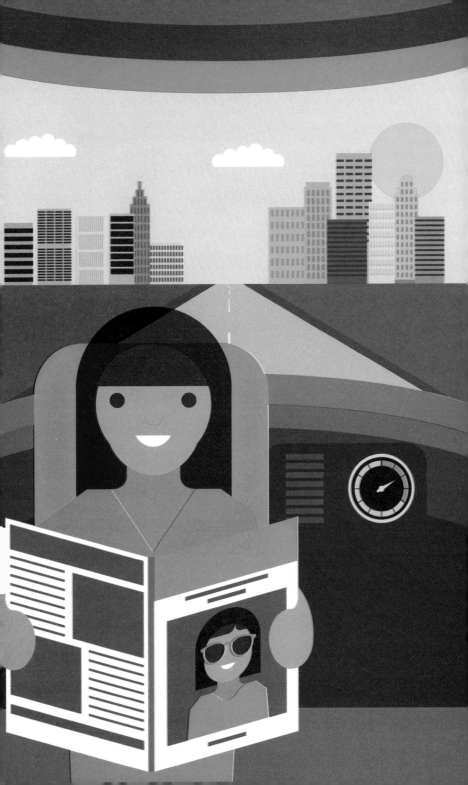

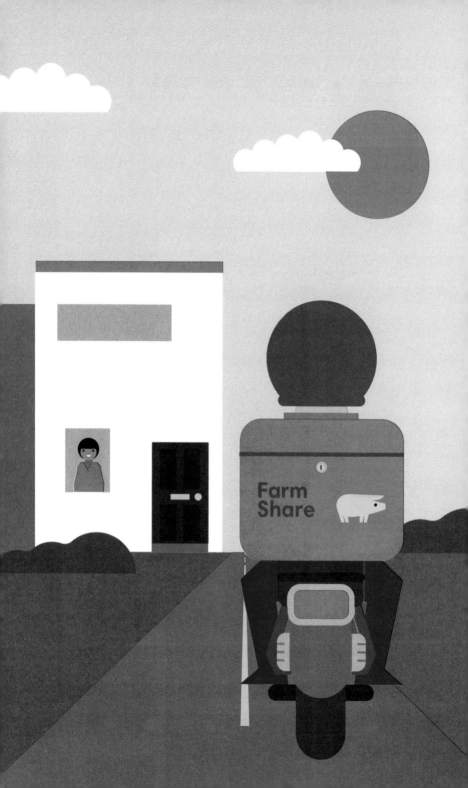

Convenient and easy to implement, home delivery eliminates the need for mobility and can make all the difference in getting goods and services home. Explore options, from online services to neighborhood food clubs and community-supported agriculture programs. Keep in mind, however, that getting out of the house remains important, and we will need to compensate for it once our lives become more convenience-driven.

Let the Food Come to You.

Put your independence to the test and explore whether you can manage your household without going grocery shopping for a week.

An exciting view from home can allow us to participate in urban activities even when we are not able to venture outside. Being able to look out of the window sounds minor to most of us, until the moment that window turns into our only connection with our context. Creating a pleasant view can be as easy as planting some new flower beds or hiring a contractor to remove a wall within the house. But if there is no satisfying solution, we should consider finding a new home, keeping in mind that one day our bedroom might be our primary living space—we need to make sure that it is a beautiful place that provides us with light, air, and a view we deserve.

Have a Room with a View.

Stay in your bedroom for a day and envision what would make your experience better, things like a new mirror, a larger window, or updates to the walls and ceiling to improve your view from bed.

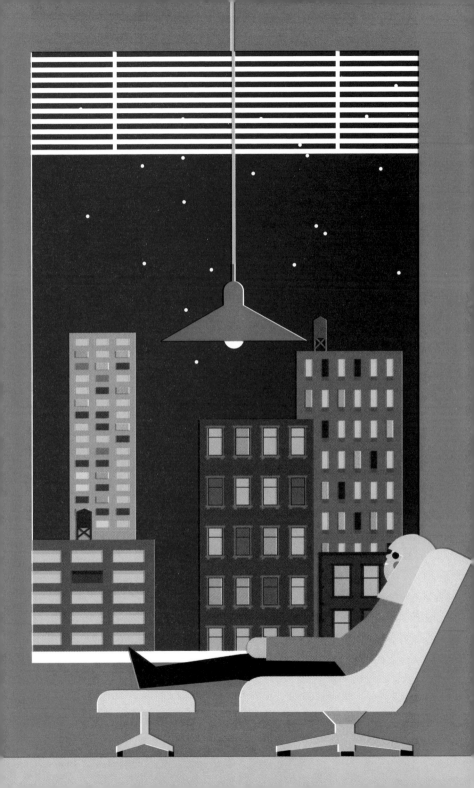

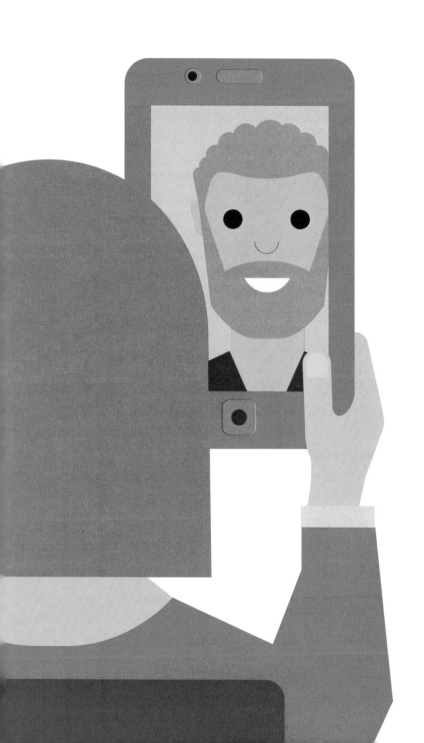

We are all used to Skype and FaceTime, but making them part of the environment beyond the computer screen has huge potential for keeping us effortlessly connected with family and friends. New technology is more interactive than ever, and can bring together willing participants.

Virtual Proximity.

Today we do not need to be next to each other to be close. Give yourself a technology upgrade by getting a phone or device that allows you to video chat with family and friends.

7

Our Homes Are Our Castles

Younger people tend to buy houses based on their resale value. The process of buying, selling, and moving is the currency of upward mobility. But at a certain moment, it is important to understand that a home's true value comes from it being completely in sync with our lifestyles and compatible with our physical and mental capabilities. Creating a good fit involves calibrating a variety of factors such as living arrangements, privacy settings, everyday activities, and personal identity. Even when we face physical or social challenges, our homes should support our needs and desires. Remember, the fundamental things that we love about our lifestyles do not change just because we are getting older.

We know that we are supposed to book checkups with doctors. We should do the same for our homes by scheduling regular appointments with an architect. The design of a home can negatively impact health if it hinders our movement or makes daily tasks difficult; an architect can anticipate the most necessary changes to the physical environment and help you plan accordingly.

Hire an Architect to Review Your Home.

Make an appointment with an architect this month and consult him or her like you would your doctor or mechanic to ensure that you are safe, independent, and at peace in your home and neighborhood.

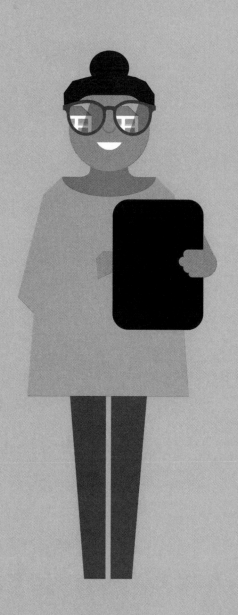

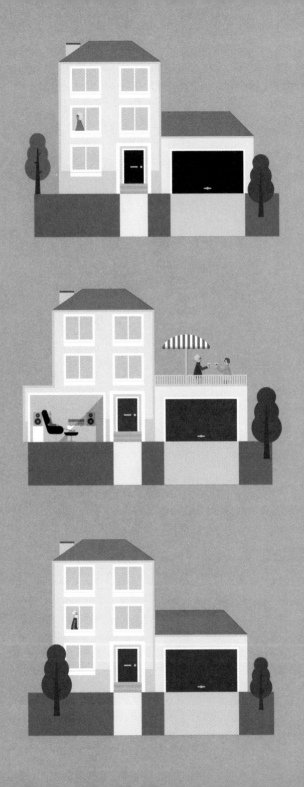

Architecture has the capacity to create peace of mind for those who experience it. Well-designed spaces can give a friendly hug, engender affection, and radiate good energy toward inhabitants. Lots of windows let the sun and views of the outdoors into our lives, and surrounding ourselves with natural materials such as wood and stone creates a more intimate atmosphere.

Make a House into a Home.

Talk with a designer and discuss materials, lighting, and color with the goal of creating a familiar environment that recharges us for the next day.

Every square foot of space costs money and effort to maintain. We need to be strategic about the size of our homes and review the areas that may become a burden in the future. We may not need the three extra bedrooms, the multicar garage, or extravagant foyers. Downsizing allows us to maintain a smaller space for much longer, and with greater ease. As a rule of thumb, plan on six hundred square feet per household member. We can all imagine ways to spend money that are more fun than home maintenance. With less to clean, heat, and repair, less truly is more.

Less Is More.

Create a list for a week of how much time you spend in each room of your home. At the end, consider downsizing to a place that has only the rooms you use on a daily basis.

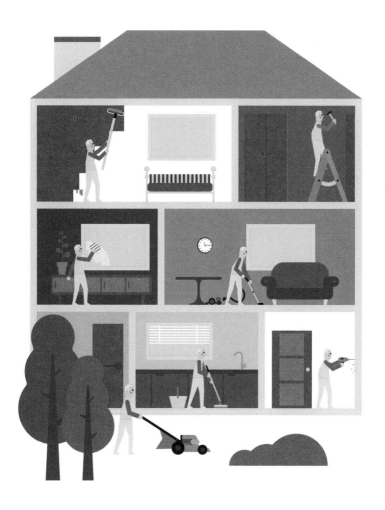

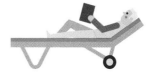

An overcommitment to "stuff" shouldn't prevent us from living in spaces of the right size. Passing things on will clean up the closets and let us have valuable conversations with friends and family in the process. We can incorporate smart storage systems and use archival photo boxes as well as digitize documents to hold onto things that are truly irreplaceable. Evaluate the things that bring true purpose and happiness to your life, then give useful items and heirlooms to family members and donate the rest to charity.

Simplify Life.

Go through a closet today and choose ten pieces to give away. Make a rule that when you get something new, you give away one thing as well.

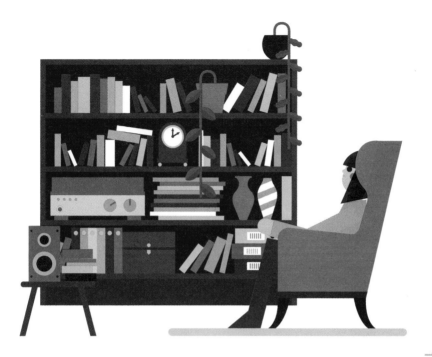

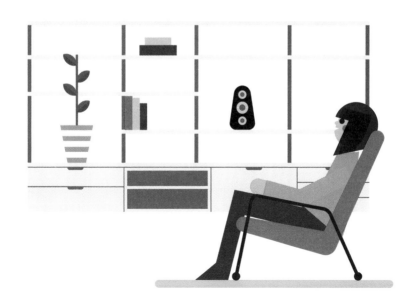

Do we really need the garden with a gardener? A pool with a pool boy? A house with five bedrooms when four are usually empty? Many of these bells and whistles are status symbols, which tie up capital and generate work that, over time, can be more of a burden than a joy. Consider how to have more amenities with less maintenance: city dwellers are already accustomed to relying on public spaces for recreation, and generally don't own much beyond what's in their apartment. We can look to this model as we scale back our housing footprint. Public or shared amenities will supply fun activities in a social setting without the hassle of ownership and upkeep.

We Don't Have to Own to Enjoy.

Map out places like community gardens, local swimming pools, and libraries that are within a ten-minute walk and start using them.

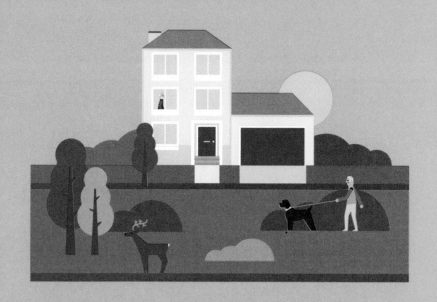

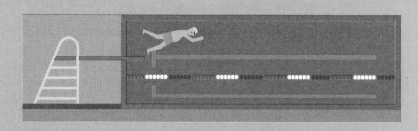

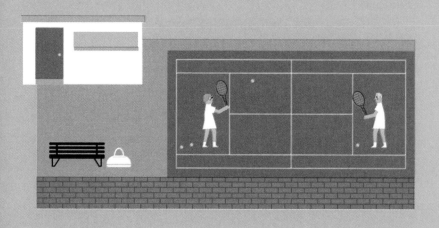

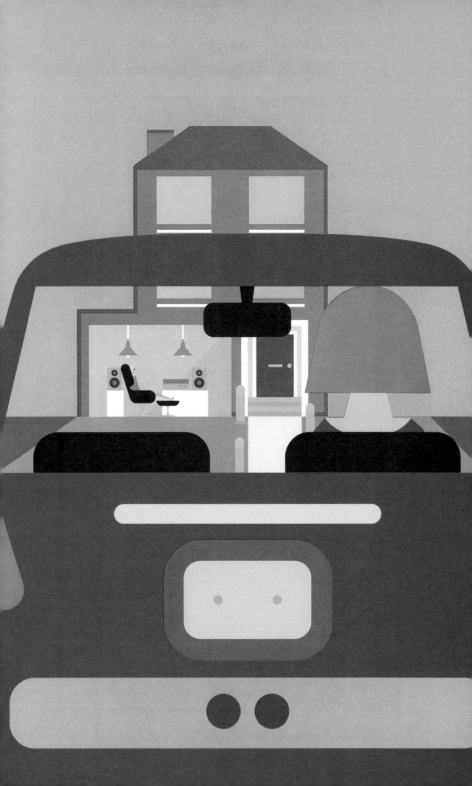

Home should be accessible from the outside in. Even in an apartment building or planned community, make sure the path you use to enter your home is simple and well-designed. Think about how you approach your house. Is there a clear, well-lit pathway to the main entrance? Can you park your car with ease, and carry any groceries or packages to the kitchen or living area without stumbling over obstacles? Improving this experience can make many aspects of our daily routine easier. Improvements can also increase our home's "curb appeal," making sure our visitors also feel welcome and can get settled easily.

Have Easy Access.

Examine your house with consciousness about how it looks and feels to someone approaching it for the first time, and improve access via all entry points with lighting and obstacle-free paths.

Our smartphones can command the domestic realm through home-control apps. With one centralized program, the phone can manage temperature, lighting, security, and entertainment systems so that the environment is truly in tune with our needs and very convenient to handle. With remote access, we can program heat so that we always arrive to a warm home in cold weather, or can turn off the pesky hallway light we forgot on our way out the door. These technological enhancements can also track energy usage so that we make smarter decisions about our utilities.

Take Control over Your Home.

Install an all-in-one interface that allows you to navigate home with just the tap of a finger.

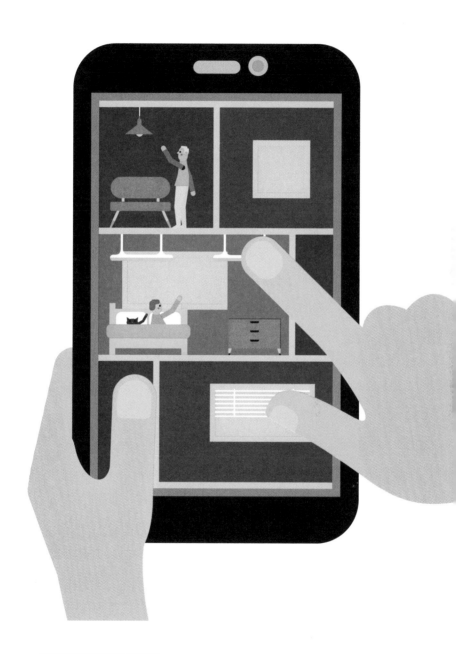

Every home has places that could use some safety improvements. Adding safety features that enhance your mobility will go a long way toward increasing your sense of safety and well-being, and will help whenever stability is in question. Installing handrails is a common way to address this issue, and if we treat them as an aesthetic opportunity, they can be interesting design elements instead of clunky retrofitted medical devices.

Hold on to Home.

Be proactive and hire a contractor to add modern handrails, door pulls, and hardware elements to stairways, halls, and bathrooms— make sure they add to the function as well as the design of your home.

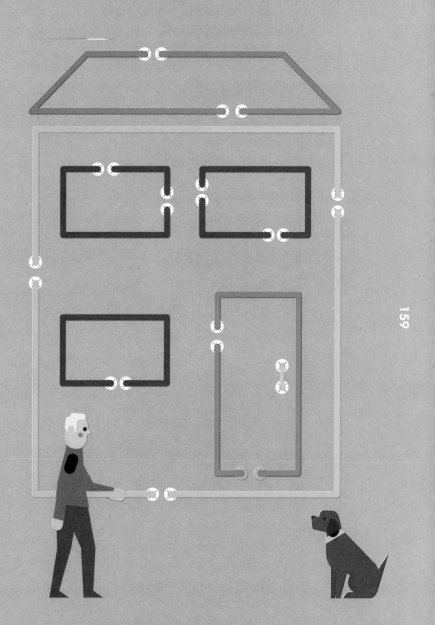

Investing in a few improvements now (and not after someone falls) will avoid more serious challenges in the future: if everyone is tripping over an accent rug, get rid of it before falling becomes a more serious danger; eliminate unnecessary transitions or changes in floor materials that could present a hazard; in places that are separated by one or two steps, replace them with a gentle ramp, and make sure all key spaces in a home are on the same floor—this means that we should be able to navigate the kitchen, bedroom, and bathroom without using a staircase. Stairs are the most dangerous site for falls that can lead to injury, medical bills, and a debilitating loss of independence. Take simple measures to minimize the chances of an accident, such as installing good lighting and handrails on both sides of the stair, and making sure treads are made of nonslip surfaces with alternating colors to make them more visible.

Create a Level Playing Field.

Take your rolling suitcase out of the closet and walk through your house with it for an hour without lifting it to test where navigational challenges may arise.

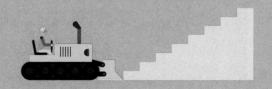

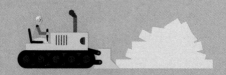

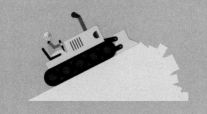

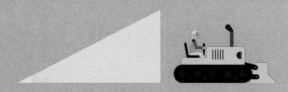

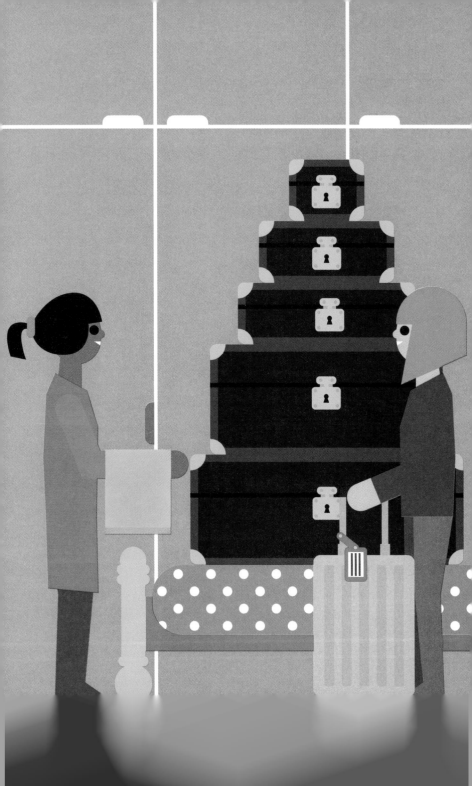

Visiting friends and family, and receiving visits, are some of life's highlights. Hotels are convenient, but having a guest room is even more convenient and reduces the financial burden on the visitor. Make sure the guest room has enough privacy, preferably with its own bathroom, so you and your visitors have maximum independence. Another bonus of a guest room is that it can become a studio apartment for a caregiver, should you ever need one.

Make Room for Visitors.

Consult a space-planning expert to get ideas about creating a welcoming guest room in your home.

Home is Where the Hearth is.

The kitchen is the heart of the home. As a center for socializing and food preparation, a highly functional kitchen can help maintain independence. Adjust work surfaces and appliances to be at the right height and configuration to work well through all stages of mobility. Editing a few details can ensure that we are comfortable and able to participate in dining and entertaining within the kitchen.

Kitchen checklist

Remember: If the kitchen or another room in the home needs remodeling to comply with these rules, do it sooner rather than later.

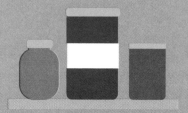

Open/visible storage; flexible pantry storage.

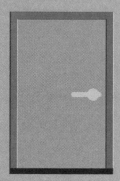

At least 36-inch-wide doorways with lever handles.

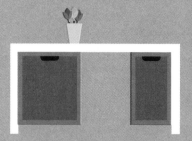

Flexible base storage allowing for use as knee space when seated.

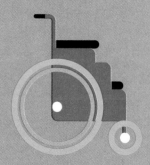

A floor made of a hard material, such as wood, tiles, or natural stone, to accommodate wheelchairs and other walking aids.

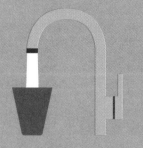

Single-lever faucets, mounted on the side of a low-profile sink.

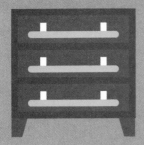

Pulls, rather than knobs, on cabinets and drawers.

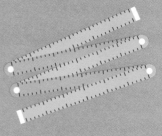

Sufficient clear floor space for work/traffic flow. You need 40-inch-wide hallways, at a minimum, to get to the kitchen.

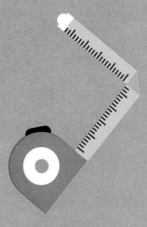

Countertops at a variety of common heights: 30, 34, 36, and 42 inches.

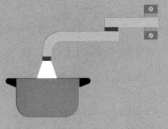

A pot-filler at the cooktop if the sink is not close by.

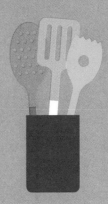

Don't forget to evaluate kitchen utensils and appliances, too. Just like you get rid of old spices and stale food, get rid of things that are difficult to use and replace them with today's modern, ergonomically designed tools. You'll have less clutter and use what you do own more frequently.

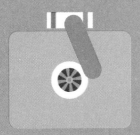

Garbage disposal mounted in the rear of the sink allowing for knee space under the sink.

Design the Throne.

We need to make sure that our homes—especially the bathrooms—are accessible under all mobility conditions and allow for easy circulation. This will keep our homes usable for ourselves and for our families and friends forever.

Bathroom checklist

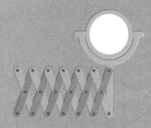

Vanity mirror at the height of a seated person or one that is able to tilt and adjust to each user.

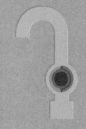

Antiscald fittings on tub and shower.

Full-length mirror.

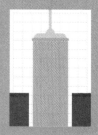

Shower designed for transfer from wheelchair (36 inches wide by 36 inches deep, minimum) or a roll-in (36 inches wide by 48 inches deep, minimum), depending on entry style.

Multiple-height vanities with flexible spaces for knees under the sink.

Create a 5-foot turning radius in key areas.

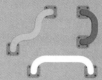

Increased use of handrails that complement your aesthetics in the toilet, shower, and tub areas.

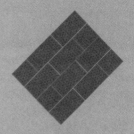

Nonslip flooring.

Easy-to-operate controls for windows, lighting, and fixtures.

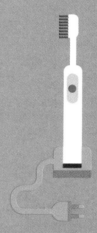

Easy-to-reach electrical outlets and controls.

Easily accessed storage at the point of use (towels near the shower, etc.).

Circulation routes a minimum of 40 inches wide leading to the bathroom.

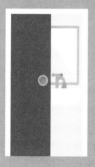

36-inch doors with lever handles and/or pocket doors.

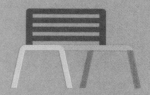

Shower chair or bench.

Sleep In.

How great is sleeping in on a Sunday morning? People spend more time in their bedrooms than in other parts of the home. In the event we have to stay in bed for an extended period of time, sleeping is not all we will do—the bedroom becomes the center of life. To prepare for all occasions, the bedroom should transform according to our needs, from sleeping to waking, and from sickness to health. Plan enough space so that a medical bed and accompanying equipment can fit, should the situation arise. We need to make sure there is a view, an easily accessible bathroom, comfortable furniture, and that we give special attention to the ceiling—remember that when laying down, the main view is up.

Bedroom checklist

Create a 5-foot turning radius in key areas.

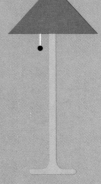

Make sure the entire room is well lit.

Keep closets organized and store things you use regularly and heavy items low to the floor.

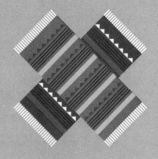

Clear pathways into and around the bedroom to avoid falls at night—no accent rugs!

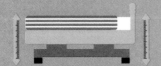

Plan for a bed with independent head and foot adjustments for easy home care.

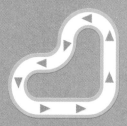

Keep a phone by the bed.

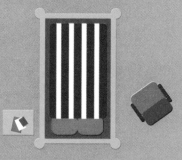

Widen circulation routes to 40 inches at a minimum.

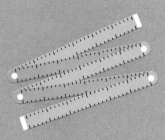

Sufficient clear floor space for work/traffic flow. You need 40-inch-wide hallways, at a minimum, to get to the bedroom.

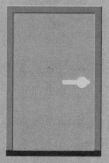

At least 36-inch-wide doorways with lever handles.

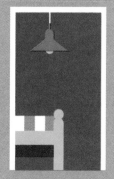

Eliminate thresholds between rooms/surfaces.

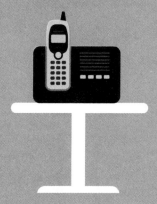

Clear a pathway around the bed so that it can be reached from three sides.

Live in comfort.

The living room is the space in which the home unfolds all of its potential. It is the place where we get together to celebrate, the place we enjoy when relaxing, and the place where most new memories are formed. Make sure the living room is designed so all activities can be peformed there, and is in sync with our lifestyle. But remember, design with social qualities in mind, since this is the place most of our guests will enjoy when visiting.

Living Room checklist

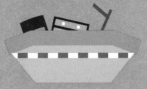

Eliminate obstacles:
Make sure there's a clear path
across the room.

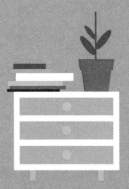

Bust the clutter: Eliminate
surfaces that are receptacles for
knickknacks or stacks of paper.

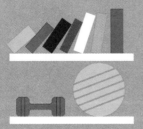

Think about multitasking: Can
this space work for your at-home
workout routine or weekly book
club? Make sure it's easy to flow
from one activity to the next.

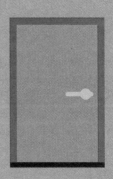

At least 36-inch-wide doorways
with lever handles.

Invest in comfortable seating. You and your friends will enjoy this room more if you do.

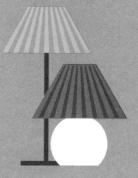

Find the light: Lighting for various moods, tasks, and times of day makes this room more versatile.

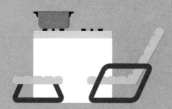

Place the living area close to the kitchen so that the person preparing food isn't isolated from the rest of the home.

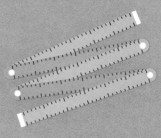

Sufficient clear floor space for work/traffic flow. You need 40-inch-wide hallways, at a minimum, to get to the living room.

Work from Home.

Consider everything we've discussed in Chapter 3, "Never Retire," and how our homes can support these goals, whether they are to run a start-up business, create an archive of our family's history, or maintain correspondence with loved ones. A home office can be as simple as a well-organized desk in another room. We can make sure that work environments follow all the rules of ergonometric optimization so we can use them whenever desired.

Home office checklist

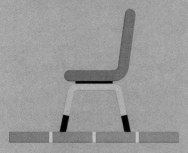

Your floor should be made of a hard material such as wood, tiles, or natural stone to accommodate wheelchairs and other walking aids.

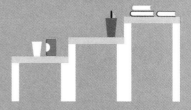

Countertops at a variety of common heights: 30, 34, 36, and 42 inches.

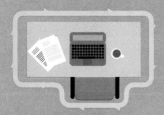

Make sure you have sufficient clear floor space for work/traffic flow. You need 40-inch-wide hallways at a minimum to get to the work desk.

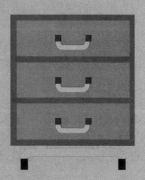

Pulls, rather than knobs on cabinets and drawers.

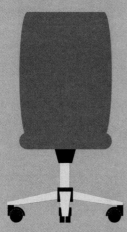

Don't forget to evaluate your chair to make it the most comfortable and productive seat possible.

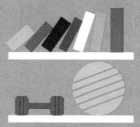

Think about multitasking: Can this space work for your at-home workout routine or weekly book club? Make sure it's easy to flow from one activity to the next.

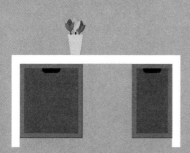

Flexible base storage allowing for use as knee space when seated.

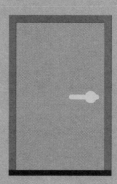

At least 36-inch-wide doorways with lever handles.

8

Add Services and Conveniences

At some point in our lives, things will get a bit harder and we will need help in one way or another. The best kind of help eases the way forward without replacing the capabilities we still have. There are many ways that help can be delivered to us: through hired service providers, strategic alliances, supportive friends, or innovative technology. These arrangements are not specifically for older people—in fact, using services that are offered in many cities and intended for users of all ages will often give us more options for less money and a better customer experience. The right help, be it a grocery delivery from the market or a ride to the gym from a neighbor, will actually make us more independent in the long run.

It sounds amazing, and it *is* amazing. Why do everything yourself when somebody else can help you with daily activities? Someone who's hired to help out can lighten the amount of tasks we have to do around the house, but also can bring a younger perspective to our day. The big hurdle is, of course, money, since employing a person means paying a salary. But there are ways to afford this kind of care if we plan for it in advance and aren't afraid to get a little creative. In some cases, housing can be offered in exchange for part or all of the care. What is good for us is also good for the economy, since employing a person also means creating a job.

Hire Help.

Contact local service listings and get information about standard rates within your neighborhood to make an informed decision about the cost of hired help.

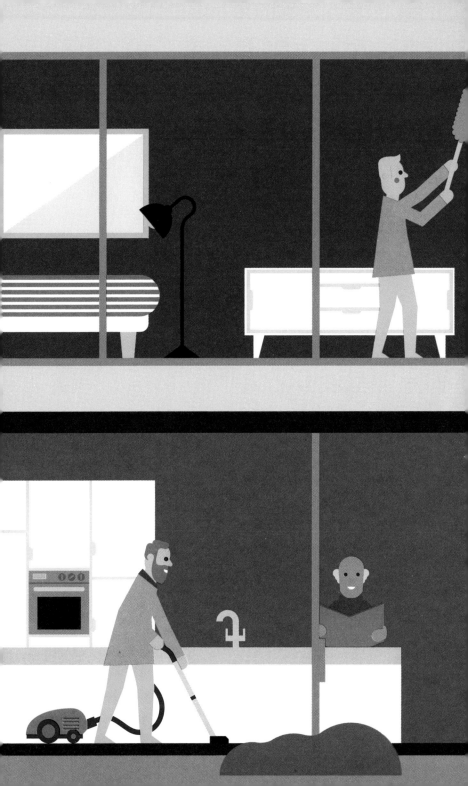

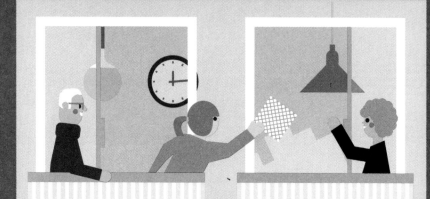
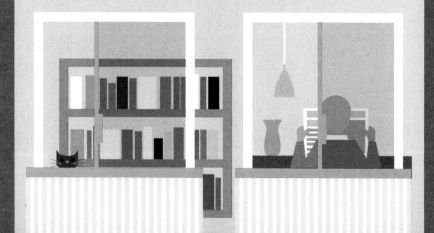

Though hiring one person for ourselves might be an unattainable luxury, we can also consider hiring one person to be shared with a group of friends. When seven friends get together and hire help, everybody is getting help for an average of one day each week. This can be enough to take the edge off some of our most demanding tasks. We also stay more connected to our friends. Strategizing about finding help can remove the fear that we will lose independence, and we'll become closer with people in our communities in the process.

Share a Person.

Talk with your friends about the possibility of sharing help as a group and make a plan about how to use the help most effectively.

The least expensive version of help is help traded with one another. One friend might own a car and be able to help with shopping; another might be a good cook who can prepare meals to be shared. Trading help is the most social of all support structures, but also the one that needs the most preparation, as well as a structure that can adapt to members' changing capabilities.

Trade Help.

Think of five things you could do for somebody else in exchange for five things that person could do for you to improve your day-to-day life.

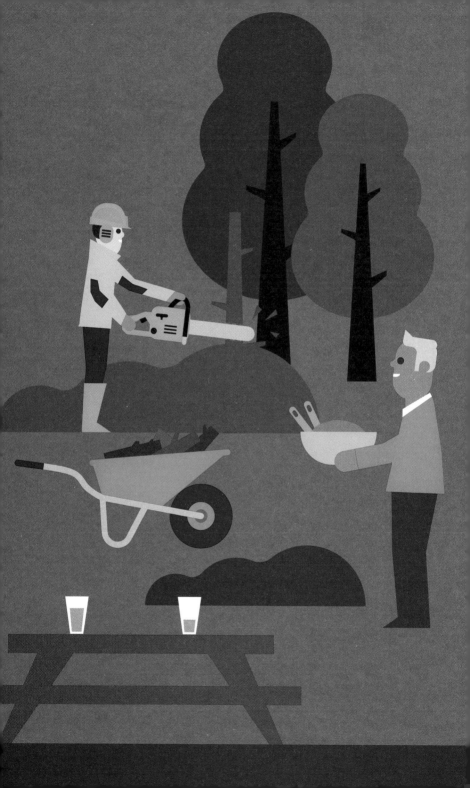

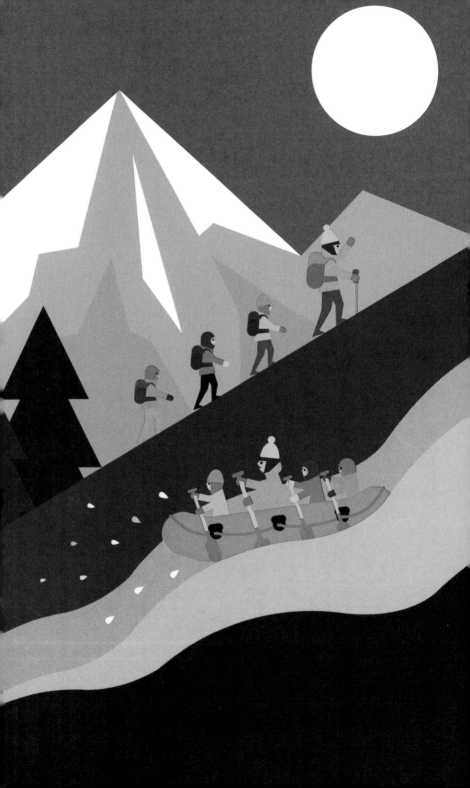

Being the recipient of volunteer help can be a beautiful experience —one that is about other people putting you above themselves. But we want to make sure that those who help us get something out of it, too. A simple thank-you, a shared experience, or an acknowledgment of relevance allows us to give and receive a currency that is not money but care. Today, when instant gratification is more important than commitment, volunteering can play a larger role.

Find Volunteers.

Search for organizations near you and create a list of ten for which you could lend a hand in the future, including your local scouting group, or a volunteer or community organization.

People like to help, but everyone is busy. The outdated model of a rigid weekly volunteering commitment can be reimagined with a more on-demand model—think of it like the DVR of giving care or companionship. This new structure can allow those in our lives to spontaneously sign up for activities when schedules allow. Make your needs known: If you know you need a ride to the doctor once a month, allow friends to sign up when they can and offer them lunch or coffee in kind.

Volunteering on Demand.

Create a shared calendar that allows people in your social network to commit to help you on a flexible basis.

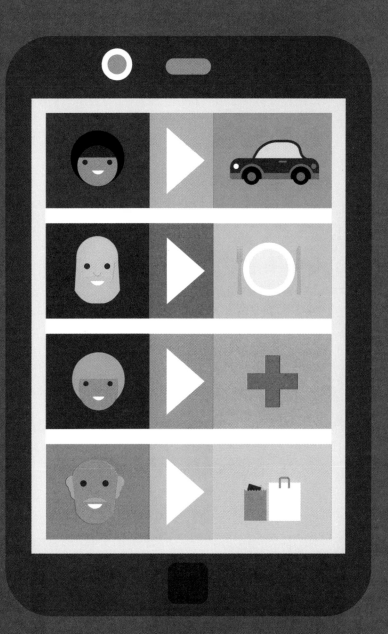

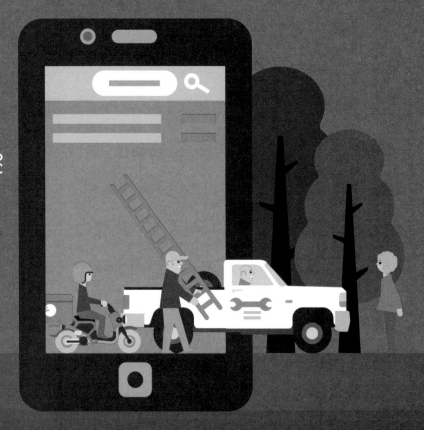

With the rapid expansion and personalization of technology, many services we never dreamed of—from food delivery platforms to chauffeur networks to on-demand housekeeping—are becoming real. Our smartphones have become coordination tools that allow us to manage all available services. There are many new opportunities that will be conquered by entrepreneurs and it will be exciting to be able to tap into these in the future. We just have to make sure that the services are easy to manage and turn out to be reliable.

Meet the Digital Concierge: Online Services.

Find favorite local services for the following:

1. Cars on demand
2. Takeout food delivery
3. Housekeeping and help with errands
4. Handymen and lawn-care providers
5. Grocery delivery
6. Online healthcare that allows your doctor to make a digital house call
7. Apps that offer personalized guides to achieve better health through fitness and meditation.

We do a lot of things without really thinking about them: brushing our teeth, bathing, using the toilet, or getting dressed. But with even a slight physical or cognitive change, these simple tasks can become burdens. While there's not yet an app to help, there are many ways to make personal care easier at any age. First and foremost, our homes need to be conveniently designed to make all hygiene and self-care activities as effortless as possible (see Chapter 7, "Our Homes Are Our Castles"). Extra help can come from family members, friends, volunteers, and service personnel.

Dare to Ask for Care.

Talk to family members and friends about the possibility of who can help with short- or long-term care, making sure to understand the extent of their possible commitment.

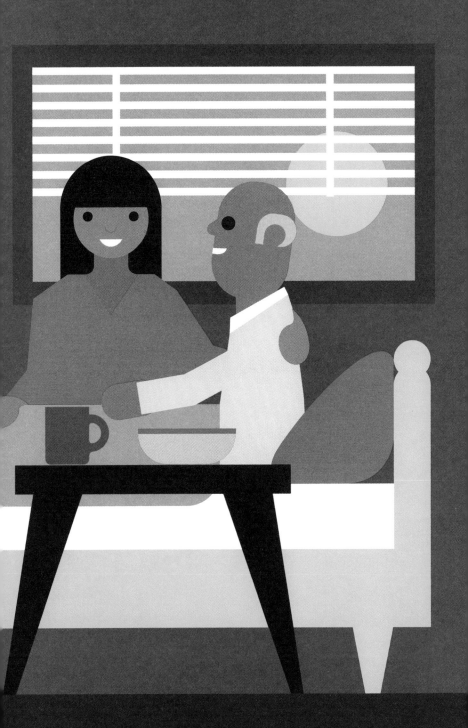

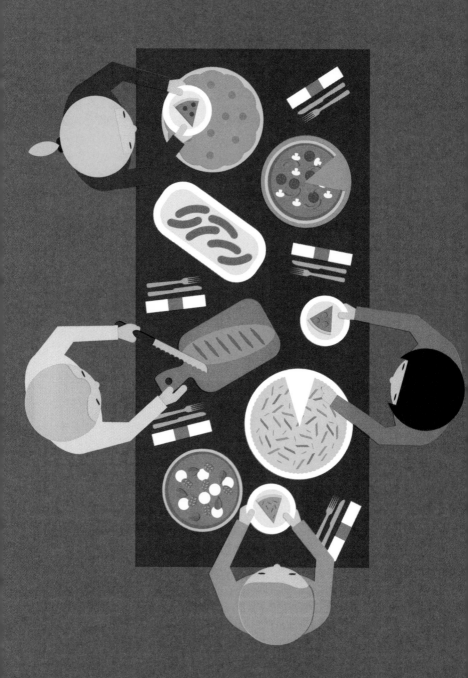

We might like eating more than cooking, but homemade food is still an economical activity that provides a healthy connection to the things we consume. Ideally, we should share cooking and cleaning responsibilities with family and friends, turning the meal into a social experience. But once this becomes difficult, we can tap into the local network of restaurants that bring food right to our doorstep. By avoiding traditional meal programs for older people that take away our autonomy, we maintain the freedom to choose what we like for dinner.

Meet and Eat.

Visit your neighborhood restaurants and ask for delivery options for your favorite dishes.

Pets are companions who join our lives and enrich our daily routines. Having animals around can cure loneliness, and provide new purpose and an exercise routine to our days. Make sure that caring for an animal does not turn into a burden. If we do have a pet in our lives, we can make sure he gets the care he needs with the help of a dog walker, a friend or neighbor willing to share responsibilities, or access to a large yard and lots of playtime.

Get Some Tail.

Try borrowing a friend's dog for a walk each day instead of getting your own puppy. This might be a good trade-off for both of you.

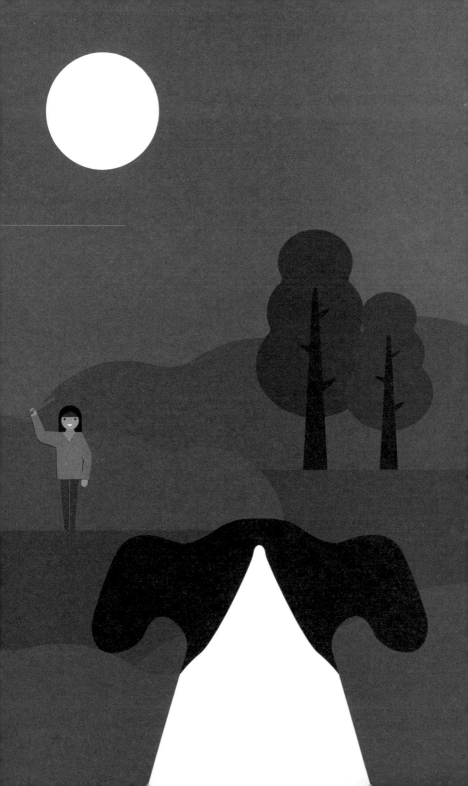

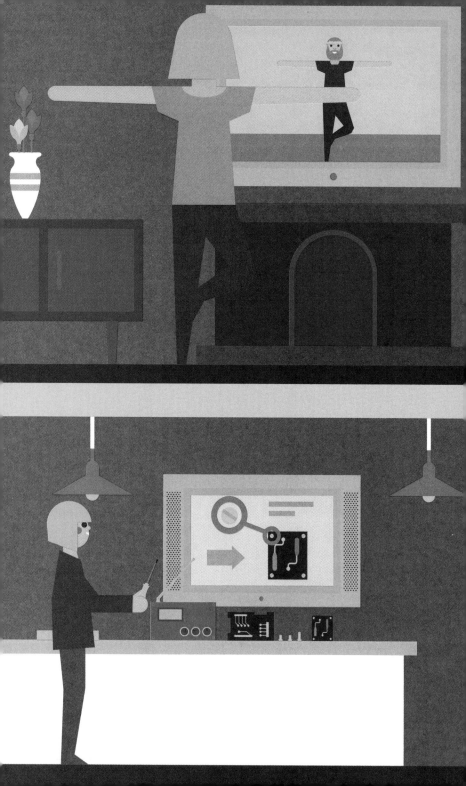

People watch up to six hours of movies and TV each day—it is part of our culture. Make sure the TV is not just on to produce white noise; instead, use it to extend your reach and experience, and as an inspirational tool. A TV can become an inspiration for activities that we have never tried before. A TV can become a resource that teaches us new things.

Let the TV Work for You.

Turn your TV on today and switch to a program that inspires you to cook, travel to a new place, or learn something new. Use TV as a service to you, not just a way to kill some time.

Having your own garden can be a joy: sitting on the lawn, enjoying the smell of flowers, and picking fresh herbs or vegetables can give you pleasure and exercise at once, which is (almost) everyone's dream. But a garden comes with big responsibility and a lot of work. To reap the benefits without the work, we can hire a gardener, share responsibilities, and reduce the size of the area we have to care for. A garden is a great amenity, but by no means essential—as with pools and larger homes, we have to make sure that the benefit outweighs the challenges.

Create Lawn and Order.

Consult a gardening expert and discuss low-maintenance options for hardy plantings that can ease your workload—or consider sharing the workload in a community garden, or moving to a place where you can enjoy public parks and gardens instead.

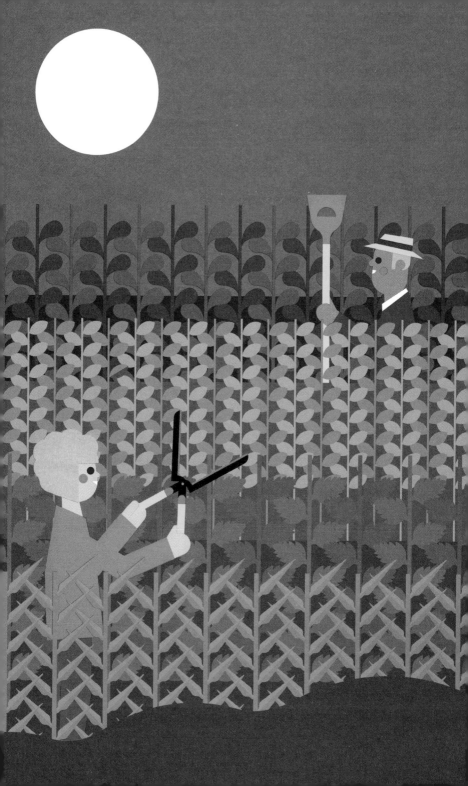

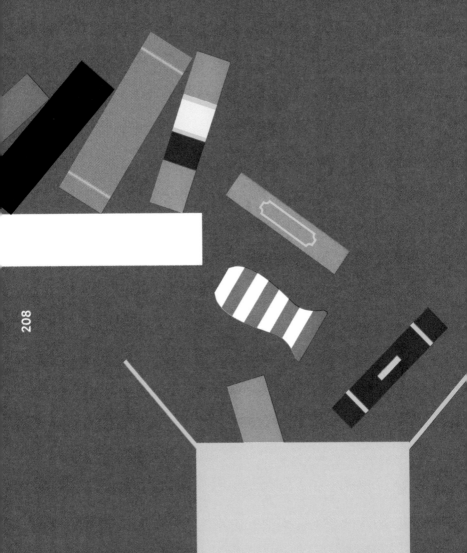

Many people think that having help with the housework is a luxury, but the reality is that thoroughly cleaning and maintaining a home can be time-consuming, backbreaking work. We could all use a little help in that area. There are many levels of housekeeping available. Look for discounted rates or volunteer services for help with general cleaning, decluttering, laundry, and minor repairs. We need to give our homes some professional attention before it becomes an absolute necessity. Declutter your life: creating a great place to hang out is not just good for morale, it will encourage friends to drop by spontaneously for a visit.

Make Home Your Homework.

Go through your closets and question every item that you have not used for the last twelve months.

Online shopping provides a continually growing level of convenience, access, and information for consumers. Many online retailers can now provide us with essentials at much lower prices than before. User reviews and prescreening allow us to learn from others' past experiences and purchase services with confidence, while search engines make it easy to compare prices and bargain hunt for exactly what we need.

Shop from Home, Sometimes.

Evaluate which products are better purchased online and which shopping trips add social value to your life. When you go out to the store today, make it a goal to chat with at least one person you meet along the way.

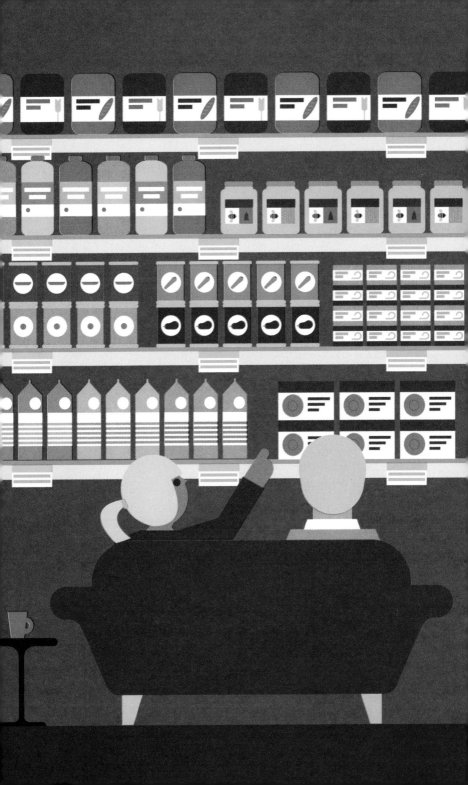

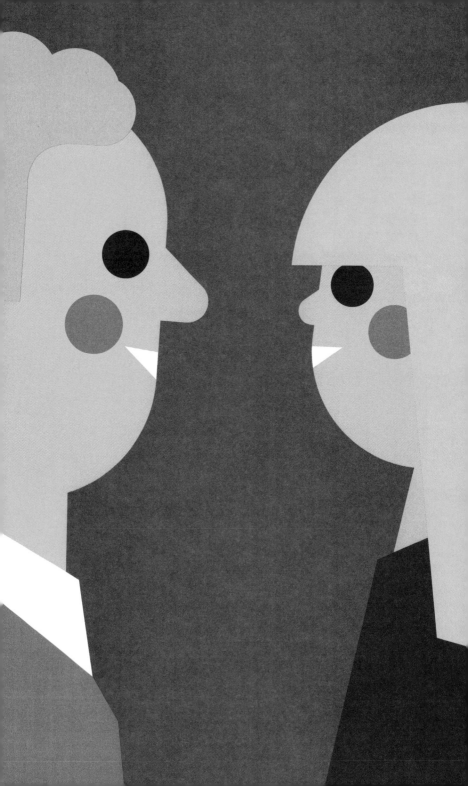

Staying in touch with our peers and communicating comes natu-
rally as long we are active and engaged. We have to make sure to
remain that way so we continue to stay connected to the pulse of
our surroundings. But not everything needs to happen in person. We
can invite people into our homes with video-chat technology, which
allows us to share a more tangible connection even when we're
not physically together. Don't forget the importance of being in the
same room, though.

Use Face-to-Face Time.

Video chat with a friend—and also set up an in-person get-together
—today.

For most of our lives, our amazing, versatile bodies compensate for difficult terrain. We run up stairs, navigate uneven surfaces, and walk for miles to a destination. We also rely on transportation like cars, trains, elevators, and escalators to help us move—but some of these tools begin to be less useful as we age. Let's eliminate the stigma of tools that increase mobility, such as walkers and wheelchairs. If we tout these tools as a necessary part of life, industrial designers and entrepreneurs might be inspired to create even newer, more forward-looking designs.

Walk for Me.

Visit a physical therapist to see what exercises and devices might help you enjoy more mobility.

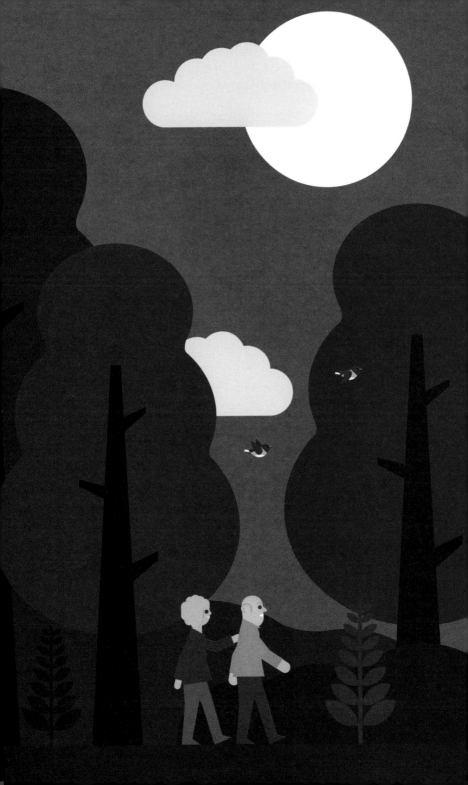

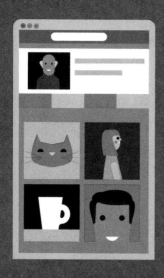

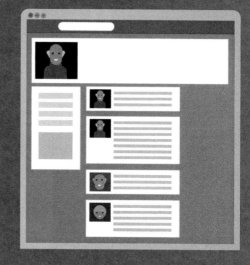

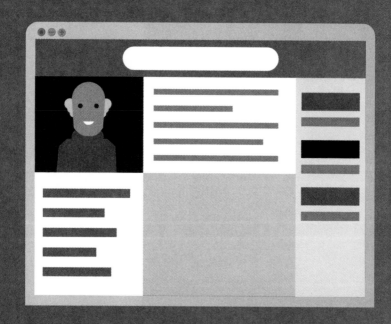

Smartphones and wearable devices are finally at the point where they truly enhance our lives, tracking activity and providing nutritional, organizational, and even emotional support. They are becoming an extension of ourselves, helping us to engage in both the real and digital worlds and bringing a new level of awareness to our health and environments. They can also become the interface with almost all of the services and conveniences we desire, as long as we learn how to use them. And we are just at the beginning of this revolution—many more opportunities to improve our lives with technology will emerge in the years to come.

Meet the Digital You.

Test out a wearable device that tracks your activity and start sharing results with friends.

Remember that all levels of medical support are available on a daily or even hourly basis; we can get the most advanced care from the comfort of home. Find a local doctor, hospital, or health-service provider and access their services from home. Nursing stations at most health-care facilities are staffed twenty-four hours a day and can answer many questions during a quick phone call, saving a trip to the hospital. Avoiding unnecessary stays in the hospital maintains a sense of independence and self-determination, even when we may have lost those things in other areas.

Stealthcare: Medical Services to Go.

Make appointments with health-care facilities near you and learn what type of care is available during house calls, then arrange for the service plan that most suits your need.

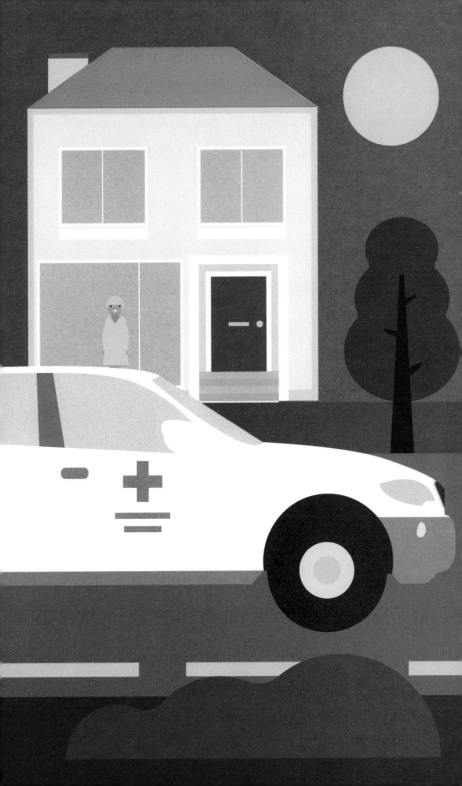

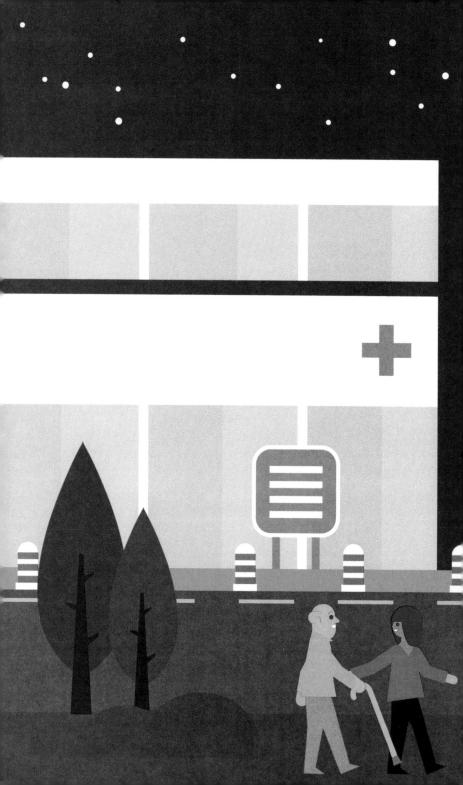

Our medical treatments and care level should be in tune with us as individuals. Go to the hospital to get back on track, but remember that there is such a thing as too much care. In fact, overly aggressive care might shorten our lives, and extend our stays in hospitals. Likewise, assisted living facilities and nursing homes don't have to be a one-way street. Make sure there is a very clear added benefit for a medical treatment and that it adds quality of life—and not just an extension to life that might be more challenging than enjoyable.

More Is Not (Always) Better.

Prepare a list of written instructions for making big health-care decisions and share it with family to ensure your voice is heard and your wishes are understood accurately.

9

Pass It On

We all are aging, but we're not alone. This is why it is important to invest in adjustments that improve our immediate experiences and that benefit our communities, and us, in the long run. Let's make the best of aging, one step at a time.

We should sit with our families and discuss the next thirty years of everyone's life. Talk about ideal living location, vacation plans, emergency procedures, and long-term health-care wishes. By introducing a sense of transparency about things like real estate, and financial and medical decisions, we will all know what to expect with one another.

Create Transparency with Your Family.

Beginning to make a plan together opens up lines of communication for every generation.

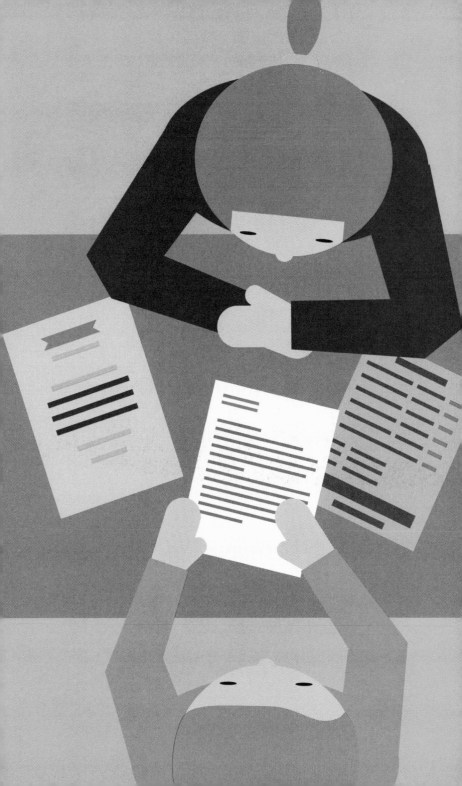

Set up a meeting with your family to discuss the coming decades and align your important future decisions:

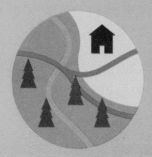

Living location.

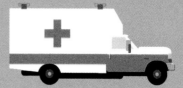

Emergency care.

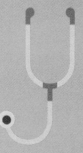

Medical care.

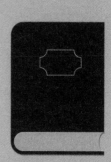

Estate information.

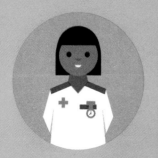

Long-term care.

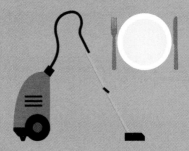

Extra in-home services.

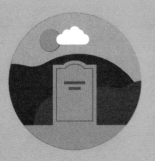

Burial location.

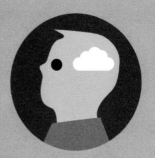

Afterlife beliefs.

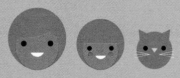

Care for children and pets.

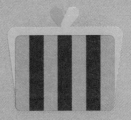

Financial information.

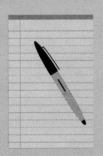

End-of-life decisions.

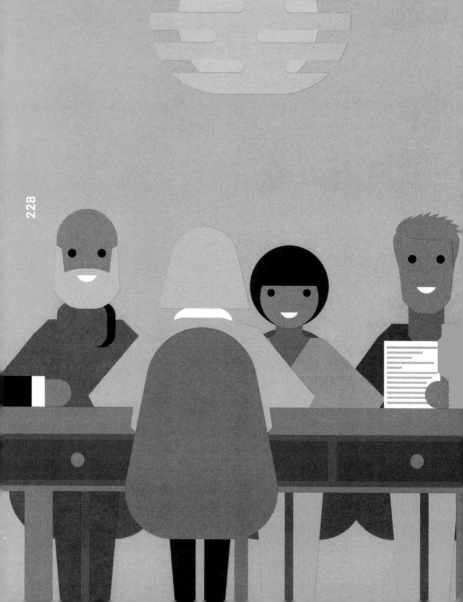

Every company and organization has a board that advises the venture about its future. This board requires companies to have the discipline to make a plan, and can be a trusted source for problem solving when complex issues come up. We can start our own board for aging, inviting four friends to become our advisors. Similarly, we can invite these friends and experts to a workshop, where we prototype the future. Share ideas with sticky notes, collages, a marker board, or with sketches—any medium that allows for a creative exchange. The goal is to find creative solutions for the things we'll encounter as we age: the concerns of home, health, and happiness. After meeting with advisors, arrange the group's ideas into one document that can be shared with all participants.

Treat Aging Like Starting a Company.

Start assembling your board and meet in person once a year. During these times, we can present visions and details about our future life, letting our advisors weigh in and help guide us in the right direction.

Once we start to live with the New Aging philosophy in mind, we can share these ideas with peers and members of younger generations. Spreading our knowledge can minimize age discrimination, once younger people understand some of the challenges that lie in the future. Teaching also helps us to put our own goals into words.

Share It with Your Network.

By using Twitter, Facebook, Instagram, and other social media platforms, we become part of a community that is helping everyone live better, longer. Share your thoughts and make a difference at www.new-aging.com.

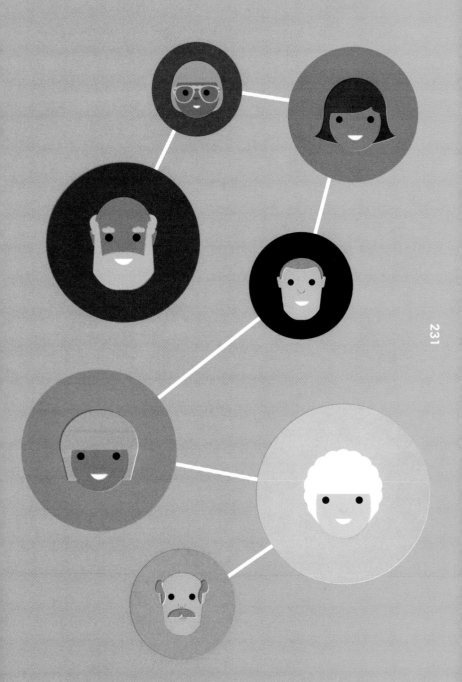

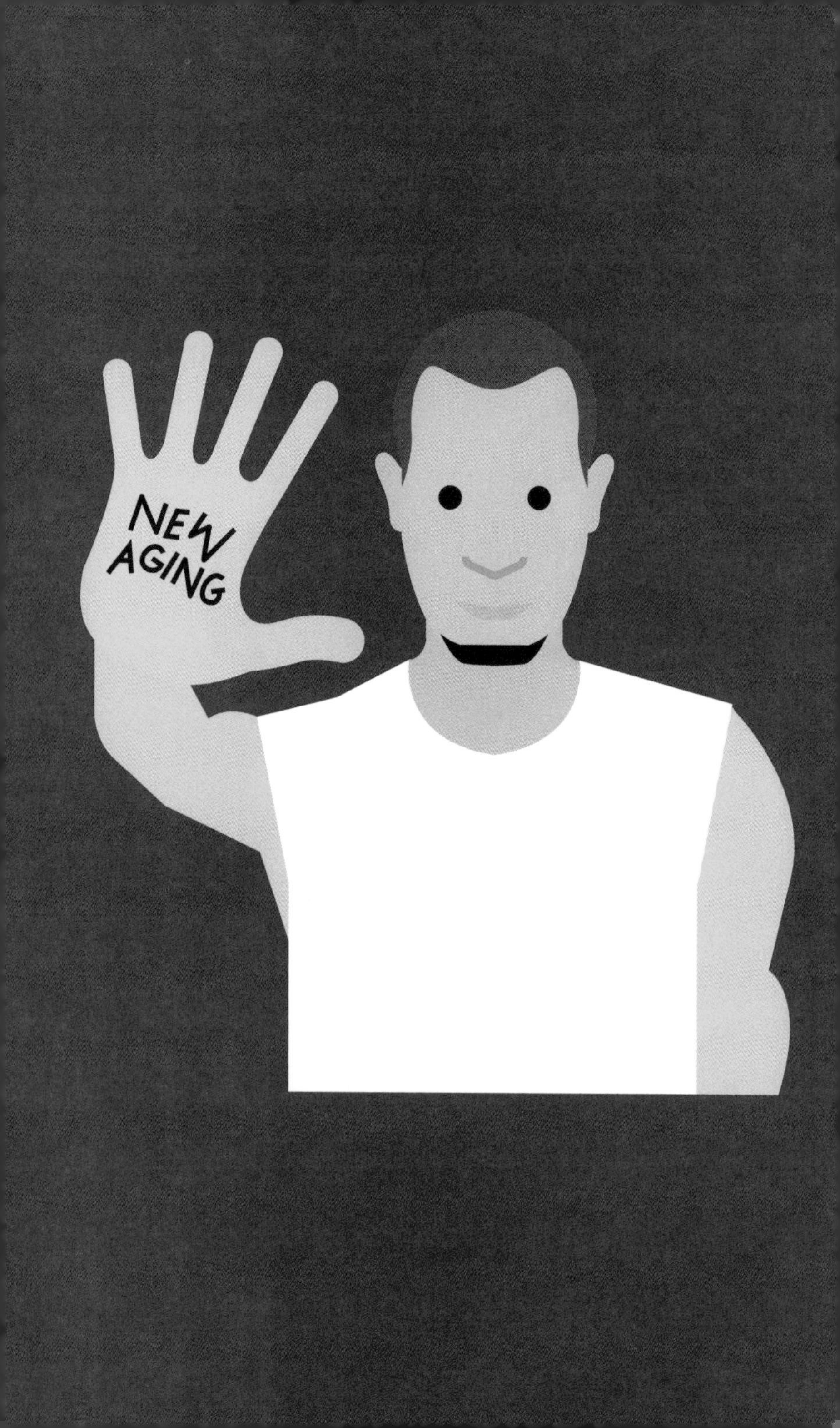
NEW
AGING

About the Author Matthias Hollwich is the co-founding principal of progressive New York architecture firm HWKN (Hollwich Kushner) and Architizer, the largest platform for architecture online.

Having previously led design teams within internationally acclaimed firms such as Rem Koolhaas's Office for Metropolitan Architecture (OMA), Eisenman Architects, and Diller Scofidio + Renfro, Matthias's architectural designs incorporate individual personality, local context, and highly social experiences and have established him at the forefront of a new generation of ground- and rule-breaking international architects.

Combining his understanding of how architecture and cities can perform better with his research as a visiting professor at the University of Pennsylvania, Matthias has developed a new line of thinking about how to make aging an empowering process. He has since shared this message at events for TEDx, PICNIC, the World Health Organization, and the New Aging conference at the University of Pennsylvania.

Bruce Mau Design (BMD) is a design firm that works with best-in-class organizations worldwide and believes in the transformational power of great design to help drive growth, engagement and awareness.

Our client partners are shaping the future of their respective industries. We work with large international corporations, visionary start-ups, expansive arts organizations, multi-stakeholder educational institutions, ambitious architects, city-builders, and governments. Our team is comprised of globally selected graphic designers, architects, strategists, UX experts, writers, and managers from diverse backgrounds.

New Aging represents the culmination of a five-year creative partnership exploring how design can help change the way we think about aging. Our collaboration with Matthias Hollwich and his firm HWKN (Hollwich Kushner) has included the development of a new community for aging populations, a new campus for one of the world's leading research universities, and a new experiment in mixed-use high-density urban housing.

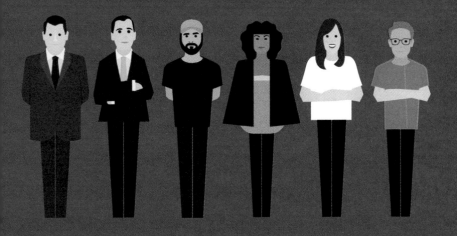

Bruce Mau Design

Hunter Tura, Tom Keogh, Cristian Ordóñez, Elvira Barriga,
Kaila Jacques, and Robert Samuel Hanson

www.new-aging.com